1996

W9-CBS-692

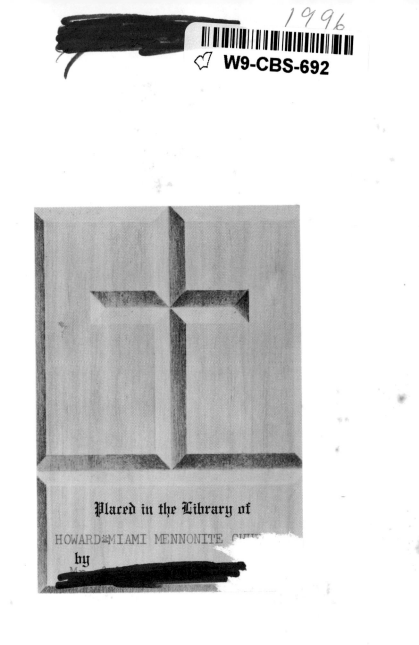

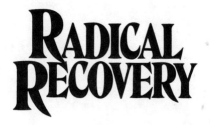

RADICAL RECOVERY

RADICAL RECOVERY

JANIE CLAUSEN

WORD BOOKS
PUBLISHER
WACO, TEXAS

A DIVISION OF
WORD, INCORPORATED

Library of Congress Cataloging in Publication Data

Clausen, Janie, 1932–
    Radical recovery.

    1. Breast—Cancer—Patients—United States—Biography.
    2. Mastectomy—Patients—United States—Biography.
    3. Christian life—1960–   . 4. Clausen, Janie, 1932–
    I. Title.
    RC280.B8C56   1982   280'.4 [B]   82–50514

ISBN 0–8499–0319–X
Printed in the United States of America

To Lee,
who gave me
the freedom to be me

and to our favorite foursome,
Steve, Kim, Candy, and Scott

Contents

Introduction

Five years ago God provided me with a radical recovery from a mastectomy. In order to cope with the psychic trauma that resulted when I learned that I had cancer, I abandoned myself to Him. What followed was an adventure I am compelled to share.

I want my readers to know that the presence and power of God is available to each of His children . . . but only if he or she supplies a necessary ingredient—belief. Human nature says: "Show me, Lord, and I'll believe." God says, "Believe, and I'll show you."

For one week I lived in the hospital, an adventure I wouldn't want to have missed. God revealed Himself again and again in the most unexpected ways. I discovered for myself what I had been reading and hearing for years: "Truly He is a God of miracles."

Not only am I writing to tell you about these miracles but about how suddenly cancer can strike. Breast cancer is the most common affliction women suffer today, health experts say. This year alone over 112,000 new cases will be diagnosed in the United States.

In my experience with both Christians and non-Christians, I have discovered that there are a multitude of lonely, heartsick marriages. Lee and I were living one of these. A

malignancy had invaded the very fiber of our relationship
and it had spread out of our control. When I abandoned myself to God at the time of my mastectomy, He performed a
miracle: why not abandon my marriage to Him? I did, and
He performed another miracle—only this one, to me, was
greater. Perhaps it was because I had lived with this malignancy much longer and it had become extremely painful;
consequently, the healing was more profound.

The healing is still taking place. Today, after twenty-nine
years of marriage, I am falling in love with my husband
again. It's as though scales have been removed from my
eyes, and I see clearly now.

For many years close friends and members of my family
have said to me, "Janie, you should write a book."

"I will," I promised, "when I have a story to tell."

Well, I now have that story to tell.

Inside of me I have lived with the gentle command,
"Janie, tell them what I did for you."

Already I am experiencing the personal satisfaction that
has resulted from being obedient to my miracle God by
choosing to write this book. It's time to begin.

1

Discovering the Lump

The week after Christmas 1976

Nearly every year, right after Christmas, my side of the family gathers in West Palm Beach, Florida, to soak up sun, pound the ball on the tennis courts, and to renew close relationships. These occasional vacations away from my husband and our four children have also afforded me much-needed space for self-examination and evaluating the progress in our family relationships.

Temporarily removed from the role of wife and mother, I benefit from the opportunity to consider myself as a woman. For ten whole days no one calls me "mom." Nothing is expected of me. No meals to cook, lunches to pack, demands to be met, schedules to follow, or conflicts to resolve.

One afternoon I was sprawled in a lounge chair in my sister Mary's backyard. The sight and scent of the tangelo trees along the canal added to my dreamy, drowsy mood. Relaxing completely, I even shed—temporarily—the ever-present stress of working with Lee on improving our marriage relationship, a firm pledge we'd made after a nearly irreparable break two years earlier. It felt good not even to think about that, just for a little while. I had brought the January 1977 issue of the *Reader's Digest* along outside with me. An article, "Heed Your Body's Warning Signals," caught my eye. I had just started reading when suddenly my senses were alerted. It was talking about breast cancer, and there was a list of things a woman should watch for: any lump or thickening in the breast; alteration in the breast's contour; any discharge from the nipple. These signals can be caused by conditions other than cancer, but a doctor's definite exam should be sought immediately, the article said.

I had purchased a vivid pink nightgown for the trip to Florida. On the last several mornings I had noticed a faint rust-colored stain in the area corresponding to my right nipple. As I thought about this, I recalled seeing a similar stain inside the right cup of my bras. I shivered in the afternoon sunshine.

"Mary," I said in a trying-to-be-casual voice, "Now it's my turn to have cancer."

My calm, low-keyed sister replied, "Don't be alarmed. It's God's way of saying that you should see your doctor as soon as you get home."

I determined to put the depressing thought out of my mind until then. But my first order of business, once home, would be to make an appointment to see our family doctor. The remembrance that I had been to see him for a breast exam and Pap smear just two months earlier was only slightly reassuring.

When I had remarked to Mary that it was "my turn," I was referring to family history. My mother had died of cancer; her mother, my maternal grandmother, had died of cancer; my grandmother's sister had died of cancer; and my oldest sister, Ruth, had survived a mastectomy which she had fifteen years earlier. My other two sisters and I secretly believed that some day we too would become victims of the dreaded enemy that had invaded my mother's side of our family.

I flew home on January 3, my skin tanned from the sun and my spirit refreshed from being with my sisters again.

January 10

My appointment with Dr. Baker was for Monday, January 10, since as secretary of the English Department at a local college I worked only Tuesday through Fridays. Our son, Steve, was a junior on campus. I liked being able to assist with his tuition and enjoyed the contact with the college students.

Dr. Baker, a general practitioner, had been our family physician for many years. A man of deep, quiet faith, he had been a source of strength through a series of family illnesses. During the past ten years my husband, Lee, had been hospitalized on four separate occasions. Dr. Baker had delivered the youngest of our four children, eight-year-old Scott. I'll never forget his gentle manner in handling Scott when he contracted pneumonia at age two months, at age four months, and again at six months. It was discovered that he had a deficiency of gamma globulin.

On that Monday morning Dr. Baker took a sample of the now regular discharge from the nipple of my right breast. A careful examination revealed a small, deeply embedded lump on the lower side of my right breast. I remember that he didn't display any sign of alarm but calmly suggested that I have a mammogram sometime during the week. He added that he would be in touch with me by phone regarding the results of both the mammogram and of the sample of fluid which he had taken from my right nipple. I said goodbye and hurried off to meet a special friend for lunch.

January 14

One of the first phone calls Friday morning at the office was from the doctor with the results of the mammogram. In his unhurried, kindly manner, he explained that there was a lot of scar tissue that showed up on the X-rays, including the small lump, but everything checked out negative. He said this was good news, that I should go on with the business of living, and that he would check the lump from time to time for changes.

Somehow I wasn't satisfied with this prognosis. "But . . . what about the discharge that is continuing?" I inquired.

"Oh, I forgot about that. I'm sorry, I've been up all night with a patient. Forgive me. Why don't you have a specialist, a surgeon, look at that?"

I asked him for a recommendation and he suggested Dr. Allen, also from the Glen Ellyn clinic. "However," he continued, "he has office hours only on Wednesdays."

I murmured a thank you and hung up.

Dr. Allen's office gave me the last appointment late in the afternoon for the following Wednesday, January 19. Unhappy with the idea of waiting so long, I mentioned that my family physician had discovered a questionable lump nearly a week ago. Could she possibly work me into the schedule any sooner? After a brief pause, the receptionist announced crisply that I would be the first patient the surgeon would see Wednesday.

A small shiver of alarm signaled from somewhere inside of me. Fortunately, our family had tickets to see Barry Manilow in concert that very evening, and the anticipation of hearing a family favorite male vocalist in person helped the day pass quickly. The occasion was memorable. Barry sang our favorites to a full house. Putting our tensions aside for the moment, I responded with uninhibited enthusiasm by holding hands with Lee and putting my head on his blue-sweatered shoulder. I was only slightly uncomfortable knowing I was being observed by the two college couples who were sitting with us. One of them was Steve and his date. Fifteen-year-old Kim and fourteen-year-old Candy were by now accustomed to their mother's spontaneous behavior. It turned out to be a perfect diversion from thoughts of malignancy, cancer, metastasis, etc.

On Saturday and Sunday I was edgy, the hours dragging by. I absorbed myself in neglected household chores. I deliberately planned a full day for Monday. At noon I played singles tennis with a friend, and at two o'clock I kept a date to play more tennis with another friend. By then the temperature had only reached the low 50s, and I had the collar of my warmup suit zipped high under my chin. Dinie, my opponent, wore earmuffs. Our breath made small circles of smoke as we ran back and forth trying to control the path of the ball. Concentrating on stroking that familiar fuzzy ball was good therapy, and I didn't think of mentioning my mysterious lump. The next time I saw Dinie, it would be under a totally different set of circumstances.

January 19

I liked Dr. Allen immediately. Coming into the waiting examining room, he greeted me in a soft, I know-you-must-be-concerned voice. I stretched out on the table and almost instantly his expert fingers located the lump. It was tucked in and under my right breast—a hard, pea-like nodule that didn't hurt when he pinched it. I watched his eyes carefully for any change of expression. I didn't notice any. Everything about him instilled trust.

After a brief silence, he said in an untroubled manner, "I don't like this lump. It is small, but with your family history, I would like to do a biopsy and make sure. My office will be getting in touch with you within the next day or two to inform you when we have scheduled surgery. If we do the biopsy on Friday, the 28th, and it checks out as a harmless cyst, you will be able to return to work by Tuesday."

"Friends have suggested that I get one other professional opinion. I would like to talk to one more specialist before going ahead with the surgery." There, I felt better having said this.

"That would be fine," Dr. Allen agreed.

Within the hour I was back at my office, launched into a busy day of typing, phone calls, faculty and students. When the opportunity afforded, I tiptoed into a teacher's office to insure privacy and called a reputable gynecologist in the Chicago area. After listening to my story, he stated in an authoritative voice, "You are taking all the right steps. I would agree to my own wife undergoing surgery with Dr. Allen if she required it."

Any reservations I had disappeared with that reassurance.

Dr. Allen's office called the next day to say that surgery had been scheduled for January 28.

2

A Biopsy

On Thursday evening Lee accompanied me to the hospital, where I was admitted after the usual filling out of forms, etc. Waiting had been made easier by the demands of getting ready for our Tennis Club party, but it was almost a relief to find my room and get settled in.

Dr. Allen had carefully explained to both of us that even if the lump looked suspicious the next morning in surgery, he would not remove the breast at this time. He planned to remove the lump and perhaps some of the surrounding tissue and send it to pathology where it would undergo extensive tests. These tests would take seventy-two hours.

In order to relieve tension, we decided to take a tour of the recently remodeled hospital. It was then that God treated me to one of His unexpected surprises.

We were walking in the lowest floor of the old wing, somewhere near the cadavers, when we heard the sound of raucous laughter. A moment later we nearly collided with two of my favorite people, Katie and Marion. Katie is my friend with whom I frequently go horseback riding. Marion is my soul sister, someone with whom I share my gut feelings. They thrust an enormous daisy chrysanthemum plant at me at the same time explaining, "What are you doing *here?* We're on our way to see you in your room and we're lost!"

Our friends went on to explain that they had just dropped supper off at our home. I noticed that the blue plaid ribbon on the plant matched the blue in our kitchen. How thoughtful. We found the nearest visitors' lounge where the four of us spent the next hour in lively, laughing conversation. There is a certain crazy chemistry whenever I am with Katie and Marion, and this was no exception—a perfect antidote for what could have been a too-serious evening.

In the morning, an hour before surgery I was given a shot to make me sleepy. Lee had arrived at my hospital room looking ruggedly handsome in a sport coat and slacks. At this important time, his strong, sensitive presence was a source of comfort. Both of our doctors were optimistic as to what the biopsy would reveal, and so were we. The daisies Katie and Marion had brought smiled at me from the table beside my hospital bed.

When they came to take me, I placed my left hand in Lee's. My right one I placed in the hand of my Lord, whose invisible presence was, nevertheless, real to me. I experienced a deep peace as the surgical cart was wheeled along the corridor into the elevator and on to the operating room. Until I was placed under anesthesia, I concentrated on imagining the figure of the faithful Man from Galilee at my side. Lee's mother, who was visiting us from Florida, had suggested this. I remembered a Bible promise in Joshua 1:9: "Have not I commanded thee? Be strong and of a good courage; be not afraid, neither be thou dismayed: for the Lord thy God is with thee whithersoever thou goest." My enormous confidence in Dr. Allen added to my sense of well-being.

Dr. Allen removed the lump and three sections of tissue. While I was still in surgery, he woke me up, bent down, and, with his face close to mine, he said, "Janie, it looks suspicious."

For some reason I was not alarmed. I simply went back to sleep.

Before I left the hospital, a doctor friend of ours, whom we hadn't seen in years, stopped by to explain the process taking place in pathology. For the next seventy-two hours they would make countless cuttings of the lump and the three sections of tissue and immerse them in different solutions before concluding whether the tissue was healthy or diseased. This particular group of doctors refused to proceed with either a simple or radical mastectomy until extremely thorough microscopic examinations had been completed. In the meantime, the patient was granted a period of adjustment to grow accustomed to the prospect of having to lose a breast. Both Lee and I appreciated this thinking.

In many hospitals, on the contrary, it is regular medical procedure for the surgeon to open the breast, remove the tumor or cyst, then send it to the lab to be examined immediately. This is called doing a frozen section. The patient is held under anesthesia on the operating table. If the tissue is benign, the surgeon will finish sewing up the biopsy incision and it will be all over. If the tissue is malignant, then the surgeon will perform a mastectomy. At the time of surgery the patient would not know if she were going to wake up with one or two breasts. Her first clue would be gained by noting the time on the clocks in both the operating and the recovery rooms. I am the type who prefers dealing with the known rather than the unknown.

I was dismissed from the hospital Saturday morning to begin the period of the Great Wait. Dr. Allen said that he would be calling at approximately two o'clock Monday afternoon with the results of the biopsy.

Saturday morning I felt strong enough to pull on my usual around-the-house uniform—jeans, shirt, and tennis shoes. My right breast was covered with a bandage which concealed

twenty-seven stitches. The area was mildly uncomfortable.
Sometime on Sunday I peeked under the dressing and was
surprised to see the rigid row of black stitches. I showed
them to our younger daughter, Candy, whose verbal reaction was "yuck."

I was tired Saturday and Sunday. I had seventy-two hours
to *think*. What if the lump turned out to be malignant? What
if I did have cancer? Could I accept the prognosis? Would I
feel like one half of a woman with one breast? Would I still
feel attractive? Could I accept the worst—what if I were to
die?

I didn't know these answers. I suspected that I would be
able to cope.

January 30

Weeks earlier we had made arrangements with Marion
and her husband, Bob, to spend Sunday evening together. It
turned out to be a timely tonic for my last evening before
The Verdict was known.

We enjoyed a long, leisurely dinner seasoned with lively,
sometimes serious conversation.

Seated across the table from our special friends, we found
our conversation shifting to the subject that simmered in my
subconscious. We talked openly about the difference that
losing a breast might make in a sexual relationship. I remember inquiring whether it would necessarily alter the in-
trinsic self that I was, sitting there that evening with both of
my breasts. Would my inner person be changed? No. I
answered the question myself. Would I be any less of a person? Again, no. But I was apprehensive. By discussing aloud
the issues I was struggling with internally I was able to face
the fact that the next day I might learn that I would have to
part with one of my breasts. I received confirmation from
Lee and from Bob and Marion that I would not be any less
whole as an individual as the result of a mastectomy. More

important than that, I would be saving my life by removing the source of the cancer. By choosing to adopt a positive attitude towards the removal of a breast, afterwards I could more easily get on with the business of living and loving and laughing.

I was wrestling with whether my femininity or sex appeal would be threatened. Would I still be appealing to the opposite sex with only one breast? Was it curves that made the difference? Past uncertainties about Lee's attraction to other women nudged my consciousness, but I pushed them down, remembering his renewed commitment to our relationship. With Bob and Marion and Lee, I arrived at the conclusion that having one less outside ornament was not of significance. Sex appeal, or the ability to be feminine, was a quality that came from *within*. This would remain intact. If I let it. Only I could control that.

And how would my husband react if there were to be a mastectomy? Would my being minus a breast make an important difference to Lee? I doubted it. My mind rested.

Having Bob, Marion, and Lee as a sounding board was of inestimable value in helping me arrive at these conclusions. By dealing with these issues *before* surgery, it would be less difficult following surgery.

On the way home I turned to my husband and asked, "Lee, do you know me well enough to predict what my response will be if I learn tomorrow that the report is malignant? I don't."

His reply was a quiet, "Yes."

"Please tell me."

"Well, first you'll cry, for perhaps a full minute. And then you'll say, 'Let's get going. I want to take the book *Joni* I'm reading, my knitting so I can work on Kim's sweater, and some note paper,' and then you'll probably ask for our bedroom clock radio."

The fact that he seemed so sure of my reaction helped my frame of mind. If he had confidence in me, then I could too.

3

The Great Wait

Knowing that Dr. Allen would be calling with the results of the biopsy at 2:00 P.M. Monday, I made plans to have lunch with a friend, someone who laughed easily and had a light touch. I didn't want to have time to do much thinking, so I left the house Monday morning to shop in a favorite store.

While dressing and driving to the shopping center, my mind raced, turning tensely this way and that. Even though I had never been particularly satisfied with my breasts— they could have been larger, firmer, fuller—on this day they appeared to be perfect. I did not like the thought of parting with one of them. They were part of *me* and had been for a long time. I didn't want to be lopsided. How would I look nude?

I was not displeased when I saw myself in the full-length mirror in our bedroom with or without clothes. Oh, I could always lose from five to ten pounds—but other than that I really didn't look too bad for a woman of forty-five. Would Lee really be satisfied with a single-breasted woman? Would I still be able to play tennis? I had been playing regularly since in my early teens. Tennis was not only an immensely satisfying form of exercise but acted as a release for my tensions. All of us in our family could enjoy it together, and I also had many special friends with whom I played regularly. . . .

The lump was in my *right* breast and I was *right-handed*. Assuming I would be able to play after a mastectomy, would I have to purchase new high-necked tennis dresses and never again wear all those pretty scoop-necked numbers hanging in my closet?

Just a minute, I told myself, you're worried about whether or not you'll be able to play *tennis* and how you'll look without a breast. You ninny! What about being concerned with whether or not there is cancer and, if there is, how far it has spread? Now that's a cause for fear!

I forced my thoughts to turn in a more positive direction. After all, the majority of breast tumors are benign. And only two months earlier I had had a complete physical exam which included a Pap smear and a thorough breast examination. "I don't think it's anything serious," Dr. Baker had told me. I continued to reassure myself. Don't forget, God has promised that he will be with me in the midst of every storm, providing strength and coping power. . . .

I tried to be brave, but fear was my companion as I walked up and down aisles of the store wanting to take advantage of the annual sale on linens. I finally decided on a pair of brown pillowcases and matching sheets for Scott's room. After getting my purchase wrapped, I drove to meet Joan at noon at a popular luncheon spot. While we were savoring corned beef sandwiches, she mentioned that she had a feeling that the report would turn out to say I had a harmless cyst. The conversation remained in a light vein. We filled each other in on our jobs and families since we hadn't seen one another for a while. I remember noticing that her low laugh was infectious, that her hair could use a shampoo, and that I loved her. At one o'clock we hugged goodbye after I assured my concerned friend that I would be okay. I promised to remain in touch.

About this time an unexplainable calm enveloped me. It

was as though an unseen Presence was whispering, "Do not be anxious, no matter what the outcome, I will be with thee."

I decided to drive to one of the women's shops in town in order to make the minutes move faster toward two o'clock. As I was browsing through the merchandise my eyes fastened on a colorful blouse with a plunging neckline. I recall thinking, no, better not. I finally decided on a safe copper-colored turtleneck shirt. I felt as though I were in a trance, every muscle and conscious thought in a controlled state preparing me to face what was to be. While having my selection wrapped, I asked the saleswoman if I might use her phone. It was time to dial home to see whether Dr. Allen had called with the results of the biopsy.

My mother-in-law, Elsie, answered the phone.

"Has Dr. Allen called?" I inquired, tentatively.

"No," was her even more tentative reply.

"Oh, come on," I insisted, "it's nearly twenty minutes after two. He must have notified you by now!"

An extended pause followed. I could hear my own breathing. There was no one else in the shop except for the kind-faced saleswoman. (I learned later that the reason Elsie hesitated was that Dr. Allen wanted to be the one to break the bad news to me.)

And then I heard Elsie's insistent voice, "Janie, *where are you?* Lee is looking all over town for you. You're supposed to be at the hospital within the hour!!!"

This was it. *Malignant! Cancer! Perhaps death!* These words crowded into my conscious mind.

"I'll be right home," I whispered into the phone.

I placed the receiver carefully back on its cradle and stood up shakily. I forced both legs to transport me to the saleswoman behind the circular counter in the center of the store. I had never met this lady but I noticed the curious look in her eyes.

"Guess what," I announced, "I have malignant cancer."

She didn't change her expression. Instead, she gazed directly into my eyes and quietly commanded, "Say 'thank you, Lord.'"

I was sure that I hadn't heard her correctly.

"I beg your pardon," I murmured.

Again. Only this time in an unmistakably clear voice. "Say, 'Thank you, Lord; thank you that I had a biopsy.'"

I followed her instructions. "Thank you, Lord," I heard myself say.

I suddenly recalled something and mentioned it. "Somewhere I have a record of a number of references confirming the fact that I should give thanks to the Lord no matter what happens. You are right. Thank you, Lord." This time, more softly.

Later I discovered the following verse copied carefully into my Bible: "Always be joyful. Always keep on praying. No matter what happens, always be thankful, for this is God's will for you who belong to Christ Jesus" (1 Thess. 5:16–18, TLB).

"Will you be all right?" There was genuine concern in the saleswoman's voice.

"Yes, I think so."

Crossing the space that divided us, she put kindly arms around me. "Let me know how things turn out."

I allowed the tears to flow as I made my way along the snowy sidewalk to where the car was parked. A sacred melody on the car radio provided a patch of comfort, reminding me that God was near. I consciously claimed His presence and His care.

As I drove the car into our driveway, I could see Lee's familiar figure through the window.

He knew me well. I walked in, and while he held me, I cried for about a full minute. And then I said, "Let's get going. I want to take the book *Joni* that I am reading, my knitting so I can work on the sweater I'm making for Kim, some notepaper, and, would it be all right if I borrowed our bedroom clock radio?"

Candy was doing homework at the kitchen table. I hugged her goodbye, assuring her that everything was going to be O.K. Then I looked into the living room where Scott was fastened to the TV. "Scott," I called, "Mommy has to return to the hospital for a little while."

Before I could continue, and without turning his head from "Leave it to Beaver," his small-boy voice asked, "Will you be back in time to take me to Glen Ayre?" This was the local swim and tennis club where he and I practically camped each summer. It was not yet February. . . . I decided not to be offended.

"Oh, yes," I assured him. I left, but not without collecting a sticky kiss.

4

What about Hypnotism?

The first thing required of me upon arriving at the hospital was to be readmitted. Lee asked if I would mind his leaving for a few hours to complete some wood deliveries while the paper work and other preliminaries were being done. I said no. He had almost crossed the spacious lobby when I remembered that I had forgotten something special.

"Honey," I called to him, "would you please bring my Bible to the hospital tonight when you come? I forgot it."

The lady who was filling my readmission forms turned and said, "I have one right here you can use if you like. It's the *Living Bible* paraphrase." (So was mine.) "Why don't you turn to Psalms 139 and read it while you are waiting?"

I did.

O Lord, you have examined my heart and know everything about me. You know when I sit or stand. When far away you know my every thought. You chart the path ahead of me, and tell me where to stop and rest. Every moment, you know what I am going to say before I even say it. You both precede and follow me, and place your hand of blessing on my head. . . .

You made all the delicate, inner parts of my body, and knit them together in my mother's womb. Thank you for making me so wonderfully complex! It is amazing to think about. Your workmanship is marvelous—and how well I know it. You were there while I was being formed in utter seclusion! You saw me before I was born *and scheduled each day of my life before I began to breathe. Every day was recorded in your Book!*

How precious it is, Lord, to realize that you are thinking about me constantly! I can't even count how many times a day your thoughts turn towards me. And when I waken in the morning, you are still thinking of me!" (vv. 1–5, 13–18).

Wow! It said it all. My spirits soared. Truly the Lord intended this for me to read. Earlier, in the car, I had abandoned myself to His care, telling Him that He was going to have to be my sufficiency. I had asked Him to make His presence *real* to me. Otherwise I wouldn't be able to cope. And I had asked Him in faith, believing that He would give me His quiet strength. Over and over the verse I had memorized since childhood invaded my thoughts: "In quietness and confidence shall be your strength" (Isa. 30:15).

When I arrived at my hospital room, I was both pleased and surprised to find Joan, my luncheon companion, waiting for me. She must have called our home and learned about the biopsy report. Discovering her there was uplifting, her presence a reminder that she cared. I remember commenting that she must have gone home from lunch and shampooed her hair. It lay perfectly, like curled cornsilk. We chatted like schoolfriends.

My sister Ruth called to say that it was going to be a rough road, that she would be thinking of me constantly, and that she would attempt to get time off from her teaching job to come out and be with me.

One friend called and then another. Word travels fast. Next Dr. Allen called to apologize that he hadn't been the one to relate the bad news. He went on to explain that he would be performing a modified radical mastectomy the next day, as we had previously discussed. With a modified radical, the breast is removed, along with some lymph nodes (the ones nearest to the breast, the assumption being that if the cancer had spread to the nodes, it would have spread to the nearest ones), but the pectoral muscles would be left intact. In other words, I translated to myself, my breast would come off, but my major chest muscle, the one that swinging a tennis racket uses primarily, would remain intact.

My dear friend Marion was the next one to call. Early in the evening Chaplain Evans from the college stopped by to talk and pray. Then my younger sister, Betty, called to assure me of her love and support. Each phone call added to my sense of well-being and to the acceptance of the trauma I was facing.

Our tall sixteen-year-old Kim, breathless from volleyball practice, arrived with her dad. Her perpetual involvement in activities at that time also included tennis, basketball, sewing, art, horseback-riding, and splitting and delivering firewood. She is a contrast of giggles and serious thinking, and that evening she wore a reflective face. Lee, more openly caring than he had been before we learned about my lump, communicated tenderness that added to my assurance that everything was going to be O.K. regardless of the outcome of the operation. The three of us read Psalms 139 together. A moment later my friend and tennis partner, Dinie, appeared. Noting that we were involved, and with visiting hours over, she said she wouldn't stay but would return tomorrow before surgery. However, she did want to ask me something. As she leaned down to hug me, she asked me to promise to be her tennis partner again this coming summer.

One more time those dratted tears stung my eyelids. I was so touched that I could merely nod a yes. And then Dinie was gone.

On a mantel at home was a trophy with Dinie's name and mine inscribed on it for being the first-place winners in the previous summer's local round robin tournament. We had finished our season with a total of eleven wins and one loss. She must have learned that the lump was in my right breast and that it was questionable whether I would regain full use of my tennis arm following surgery.

February 1

Early Tuesday morning our family physician strode into my hospital room to announce that surgery would be between 5:00 and 6:00 P.M. His manner was quiet and reassuring. As we were chatting, an idea occurred to me. "Dr. Baker," I asked, "would it be at all possible for you to hypnotize me before surgery? I'd like to try for the same kind of positive experience as when you placed me under hypnosis while I was in labor with Scott." That had been a highly effective method of relieving discomfort, I'd found. Many people are concerned about hypnosis, and I was also. However, Dr. Baker, one of the rare, old-fashioned general practitioners, has a unique ability to inspire confidence. His reputation is above reproach. I trusted him implicitly, as did countless others.

Two things are necessary if a person is to be placed under hypnosis. One is that he *wants* to be hypnotized, and the second is that he has absolute confidence in the person doing the hypnotizing. I qualified on both counts. Hypnosis doesn't cure, but it relieves pain and enables one to heal more quickly. It is one way to approach the problem of pain, especially for a patient who has a tendency to become uptight.

I think it is important to note here that I *wanted* to be hypnotized. *I wanted to be free of pain*. Motivation was a significant factor in enabling me to cooperate with Dr. Baker and thus be fully hypnotized. I wanted to have a radical recovery from my mastectomy in order to return to my world of living and laughing and loving.

Replying in her newspaper column to a concerned reader, Joyce Brothers commented that there is nothing especially frightening or mystical about hypnosis, nor is it necessary to use any object or gadget such as a dangling watch in order to induce a trancelike state. No one can be hypnotized if he or she doesn't want to be, nor can anything be created in the hypnotized person that didn't exist before, she said. Rather, the hypnotized person is in a state of intense concentration, in which the mind (about 10 percent conscious and 90 percent unconscious) is extremely open to suggestion. Smoking, nail-biting, overeating, unreasonable fears have all been controlled in many persons through hypnosis, and it can even help lower blood pressure.

On this Tuesday morning, the day of surgery, Dr. Baker agreed to hypnotize me. We decided to go ahead right then. By this time Lee had arrived, so he, too, witnessed the following scene:

Dr. Baker began to talk to me in a soft, soothing manner, telling me to relax and that I would soon begin to feel very sleepy. He picked up my right arm and told me that it was heavy, extremely heavy, and then he released it, allowing it to fall freely on the bed. He said that it was important that I not try to help it but rather allow it to fall by itself. He then did the same thing with my right leg.

He continued in this manner with my left leg, my left arm, and lastly, my head. His voice remained consistently quiet.

He then told me to imagine that I was seated under a tree by a still, blue lake. There was not a single ripple on the lake. "Do you see the lake?" he inquired.

"Yes," I murmured.

I did my best to concentrate on following his instructions. The doctor then described a small, log cabin that could be seen across the lake. Again, he said, "A small log cabin can be seen across the lake."

I noticed that he said everything twice . . . probably for emphasis. "Do you see the cabin?"

I saw the cabin.

He then told me that if I looked closely, I could see small

puffs of smoke coming from the chimney and drifting lazily into the clear blue sky. He continued in a drowsy drone, "Puff, puff, puff." His voice faded on the final "puff."

With concentrated effort I saw the small log cabin across the calm blue lake in my imagination. I even saw the puffs of smoke drifting lazily into the sky.

When I was in a trancelike state—a state of intense, aroused concentration—the doctor made the following suggestions to my subconscious mind: You will awaken this evening following surgery with no nausea and a slightly hungry feeling. You will have a minimum of discomfort, and you will have good use of your right arm. He spoke slowly, quietly, and with emphasis. He repeated each suggestion twice. I believed, as I was hearing his voice.

An amazing thing. During the period of hypnosis the phone remained silent. As soon as Dr. Baker brought me out of the hypnotic state, it began to ring. For the rest of the afternoon, it couldn't seem to stay quiet long enough for me to have an uninterrupted conversation with the friends who kept coming in.

Dinie arrived looking lovely in a striking color combination of black and camel, her blond hair smoothed into a perfect pony tail. Marti came and presented me with a poem that she had composed and an evergreen planted in a clay pot:

For Janie . . .

Oh, God, creator of this tiny tree
    that weathers every storm and changing season,
    that sways and bends in wind, but does not break,
    and firmly stands, its needles fresh and ever-green . . .
Keep Janie rooted in Your constant Love
    and though she cannot understand Your reason,
    sustain her now, though buffeted by winds of pain . . .
    tend, nurture, and restore her by Your creator-hand unseen!
                                        Love and prayers . . .
                                        Marti

Just before two o'clock, Marion arrived and told me that she loved me very much. We had hardly begun to chat when two young men wearing white appeared in the doorway. They were pulling a cart. They explained that they were here to *take me to surgery!* I was not prepared for them. It couldn't be. Suddenly two nurses walked briskly into the room carrying that loathsome hospital gown and a needle, my presurgical shot. Everyone appeared to be in a hurry.

"Come on, Mrs. Clausen, let's get into this gown; I'm going to give you your shot. Let's get to the bathroom. We're taking you to surgery now."

I objected. "I'm sorry, I'm not going. My doctor said that surgery would be between five and six o'clock. My husband is delivering firewood. I am not going."

I turned to Marion, determined to ignore the intruders, and attempted to continue our conversation.

"Come on, you have to go. Now lie still so I can insert this needle."

"Listen," I protested, "last week they came an hour ahead of time to give me my presurgical shot. I was able to get used to the fact that I was about to have an operation."

I discovered then what I had already suspected. One doesn't tell hospital personnel that one isn't ready to have surgery. When they come for you, you go.

"Marion," I pleaded, "please get Elsie on the phone and see whether she can locate Lee. And, oh Marion, we hardly had a chance to be together . . ."

The cart was moving out of the room and I was on it. The last thing I remember seeing was Marion picking up the phone to dial, and then she disappeared from sight.

5

Journey under Protest

We were heading toward the elevators that lead to the operating room. I could feel myself giving in to the inevitable effects of the shot I'd just been given. In between spurts of anger at God for letting this happen, scenes from my past played in my altering consciousness . . .

. . . *I was a young girl of twelve again, growing up in the picture postcard countryside of Chester County, Pennsylvania, with its gurgling streams, fields of buttercups, and myriad mock orange and rose of Sharon trees. Sitting in our family pew alongside my mother, sisters, and brother in the handsome gray stone church where daddy preached, I felt loved and secure. Being there was as natural as breathing, and our parents' strong faith radiated into all our lives. The light streaming through the stained glass windows imparted a sense of grandeur while the majestic tones resounding from the organ enhanced the new intimacy I felt with Jesus as my Savior and Friend. Welling up within me was the same tremendous spiritual emotion I'd experienced just a few weeks earlier when I'd made my commitment to Him. . . .*

With the sound of the elevator doors closing and the hum of the motor, my frustration burst forth all over again. How dare the hospital do this to me? I began to argue with God.

"You promised that You would be with me. You know how

much I need Lee at a time like this. I'm about to have my breast removed and he's not here. Why have You allowed this to happen? Where are You? Why have You failed me?" . . .

My thoughts swirled to Lee . . .

. . . *Lee,* . . . *Tall, blond, good-looking, he'd been introduced to me at a roller skating party at Wheaton in March of my freshman year. "Oh, so you're Mary Woll's little sister," he teased. "Say small ball." I did, and he laughed aloud. Those who have spent most of their lives in the Philadelphia area have a distinct way of pronouncing the sound "all." I labeled him as a tease and an unusually smooth skater.*

A few weeks later my roommate and I were studying in the library. Lee and a buddy approached our table and inquired whether we wanted to get a bite to eat. I was just finishing the last of my hamburger when Lee turned to me and asked, "Do you have any money with you? You ate more than I had planned." I had been right about the teasing.

There was more. The four of us were assembled in Don's car and on our way to the dorm when Lee announced from the back seat (next to me), "Janie, stop trying to hold my hand. This is the first time we've been together!"

I was embarrassed. At the same time, I liked it.

We were married four years later, December 19, 1953, in an elegant evening event. My father escorted me down the aisle and then stepped forward to perform the ceremony. The bridesmaids—my three sisters and Lee's sister, Jeanie—wore crimson and green velveteen dresses and carried white and red poinsettias. The church was festive with fresh greens and banks of poinsettias softened by the glow of candles. It was a wondrous Christmas celebration. A touch of sentiment was added when Lee sang to me at the reception. . . .

The elevator doors opened to receive us, the white-clad figures pushing my cart in unceremoniously. I continued my argument with God: "Four days ago when they came for me I was psychologically prepared. Lee was beside me holding my hand as we walked along. In fact, You held my other hand. I knew what time to expect to be ready and that's when they came. Do You expect me to have perfect peace and a quiet center now? And You know how upset Lee will be when he discovers they took me way ahead of time."

The figures with their walking white legs guided my cart inexorably toward its destination.

"Well, You did promise that when I passed through the waters You would be with me. Perhaps You want me to face this with You—You alone. Maybe I shouldn't have to have Lee with me. I will try to trust You. . . ." Another wave of memory washed over me.

. . . *It was a hot, bright summer afternoon in 1965, and the whole Woll clan had gathered for its annual vacation time together. Across the sparkling waters of Bass Lake I could see my oldest sister, Ruth, swimming in slow circles around Lee. He was obviously tiring in his effort to reach shore on the far side. He'd challenged Ruth to a race, not expecting her to accept, let alone humiliate him, but he hadn't reckoned with her fierce competitive spirit. She was determined to show she'd completely and quickly recovered from two recent operations—a radical mastectomy of the left breast and a subsequent hysterectomy, all at age thirty-five. She'd reached shore when he was only halfway across, then dived in and returned to provide him a precautionary escort. Admiring her, I hoped I had a big chunk of that Woll family determination too.*

My jumbled thoughts churned on, forming a collage of images . . .

. . . *My next older sister, Mary, losing her daughter, Bonnie Sue, in a drowning tragedy, but standing firm in her faith. . . . Our younger sister, Betty, horribly injured in a near-fatal auto crash, both legs crushed, spine fractured.*

Coming into focus was our first meeting after her recovery. We were meeting her plane at the tiny airport in Eagle River, Wisconsin. I was wearing dark glasses so she wouldn't see my tears when I got my first glimpse of her with only one leg. Tall and willowy, wearing a miniskirt, she appeared in the doorway of the plane and gave us a bright, saucy wave. After a hug and a hello, we ushered Betty into the back seat and were on our way to the rest of the waiting family back at the cottage. Suddenly, a mesh-stockinged artificial leg appeared over the top of the front seat between Lee and me. It was accompanied by a matter-of-fact command, "Now, don't feel uncomfortable. Take a good look at this thing, because we are all going to have to learn to live with it. . . . And, don't forget—if you walk out into the street without looking to see if a car is coming, you'll get hit like I did."

Images continued to form. . . .

. . . Betty, playing tennis again, trying to regain her championship form . . . dancing at the Nixon Inaugural ball . . . learning to water-ski . . . accepting the Philadelphia Sports Writers Association Award as Most Courageous Athlete of 1968. . . .

We had arrived. The area was dark and depressing. My cart was the last one in line. Ahead were mysterious-looking double doors. I was cold. And frightened. And mad. And disappointed. A person in white handed me a warm cotton blanket. It felt wonderful against my skin—like it was fresh from the oven. I learned later that it was. Blankets for surgical patients are kept warm in a special warming oven.

I concentrated on trying to relax and to allow the Spirit of God to be my sufficiency. My confused thoughts continued.

"Well, Lord, I know what I'll do. I'll help You. With me helping You, perhaps we can get Lee here."

I turned to the nice young men standing by my cart in that dimly lit hall. Having a son their age made me feel comfortable with them. "Say, would you do something for me? There's a possibility that a red-faced, blond man might be rushing into the hospital right about now. Would you go to the lobby, see whether you can intercept him, and tell him where I am?"

"Sure. I'll be glad to," murmured one of the boys.

I turned to the remaining lad. "Would you return to my room on the fifth floor in the new wing and see if my husband is there? He won't have any way to know which operating room you have taken me to."

Another ally had been engaged.

I practically willed Lee to be on his way to me, and at the same time tried to face the fact that he did not intend to come to the hospital until late afternoon.

And then I noticed two things. First, there were no carts between me and the mysterious double doors, and second, a familiar figure was walking toward me. It was Dr. Allen.

"Hi there, Janie. Ready to go in?"

"I'm trying to be," I answered bravely. "The problem is that Dr. Baker said that surgery wasn't scheduled until five or six o'clock and Lee is busy making wood deliveries."

"I'll be your Lee," Dr. Allen volunteered in a soothing, resonant voice. He reached for my left arm and began stroking it.

"That feels good. But . . ." and I hesitated, "it doesn't feel like Lee."

"I'll tell you what," Dr. Allen continued, "I'll make a couple of phone calls, and if Lee's not here by the time I've finished, we'll go in."

"O.K.," I agreed reluctantly.

I watched his retreating form until it became a shadow at the end of the hall.

"Please, Lord, I know You have the power to make Lee appear this very minute. You parted the Red Sea. You closed the lions' mouths for Daniel, and You can do this for me."

I was pleading now.

Still no sign of Lee or the young boys who went to find him.

I gave up—surrendered my will to let go of the condition that Lee *had to be with me*. Dr. Allen reappeared and said kindly, "Let's go."

I was wheeled through the double doors into a brilliantly lighted room decorated with a team of white-clad figures, complete with white masks. *This was it*. I relaxed with the knowledge that my God was with me.

A pleasant faced anesthesiologist asked, too brightly, "And how are you, Mrs. Clausen?" For some reason I resented his cheerful, matter-of-fact manner. How many times each day he must ask this of the victim he was about to put to sleep, checking the chart to learn each name. The question appeared to be artificial. I watched the needle poised in his hand as he searched my left wrist for a prominent vein in which to insert the pentathol.

Then it happened. A sudden clamor could be heard in the expectant hush of the operating room. A loud, angry voice shattered the silence. Instantly, I identified its owner.

Lee was shouting now. "You can't operate on my wife! She's about to have a major operation and I haven't been with her. There is no way I'm going to allow you to put her to sleep!"

Silence.

6

Where Was Lee?

The nurse was the first to speak. "The patient's husband is here," she explained to Dr. Allen. "He is extremely angry that he hasn't been able to be with her before surgery. He is insisting on seeing her!"

Silence again . . . deafening. I felt as though I were part of a live television drama.

Then in a calm, quiet voice, but with authority, Dr. Allen said, "Wheel her out to the corridor. She and her husband may have ten minutes alone."

Wow. And to think that I was trying to help God make this happen. He didn't need me. What He did need was for me to trust Him.

I was wheeled out of the operating room, past two sets of double doors, and into a crowded corridor. And there was Lee.

During the next ten minutes Lee held my hand, put his face close to mine and talked quietly to me. He told me that he loved me very much and that he was proud of me. He assured me that he was never going to allow them to operate unless he was there with me. Not being a man given to making verbal declarations of love, his words sounded like sunshine. I was surrounded with a strong sense of his support. I felt comforted and cared for. Those ten minutes were per-

meated with closeness and a delicious feeling of together-
ness. They will linger long in my memory as an unexpected
and generous gift from God.

I was overwhelmed with how God had worked things out
and the tears were wet on my cheeks. He knew all along that
Lee was going to make it to the hospital in time to be with
me. I think He simply wanted me to be willing to face
surgery with His presence alone. And, because I finally got
to that place, He rewarded me with the gift of my husband's
presence.

From time to time I have noticed that when I truly attempt to obey God, and to do His will, He lets me know in
some small way that He is pleased. It's as though He smiles,
and then sends me a thank-you surprise.

Later Lee told me his part of the story of that early afternoon.

In winter, to compensate for the lull in the landscaping
business, Lee carries on a brisk business in firewood, February being the peak of the season. Concerning my impend-
ing surgery, he had peace of mind that everything would be
O.K., as I did; he felt good about the eventual outcome of
the operation. So, the morning of the day for surgery, when
Dr. Allen informed Lee that it would not take place until
6:00 P.M., he left the hospital to make wood deliveries. At
1:00 P.M., before leaving with another load, he decided to
check with his mom to see whether I had called with any
new information. She informed him that she hadn't heard
anything. He mentioned that he would be gone about forty-
five minutes on a delivery in the south Glen Ellyn area.
Calling again from there, Lee was informed by Elsie that
she had just hung up the telephone from talking with
Marion. They were taking me to surgery.

Lee frantically heaved the wood from the truck into the
garage and shouted to the puzzled customer, "I must leave
immediately."

He drove home, quickly changed clothes, and hurried to

the hospital. He headed immediately for my room on the fifth floor in the new wing, the last room at the end of the hall. He never stopped running or took time to remove his topcoat. Upon entering my room, he noticed that the bed was made and I was gone. He raced for the elevator, yelling as he passed the nurses' station, "Where is the operating room?"

Someone answered, "On the third floor."

He hit the down button, bolted through the elevator door, and was soon on the third floor. He passed another nurses' station and was directed, "At the end of the hall, turn left and then right."

At the end of the hall he was met with closed double doors and a sign OPERATING ROOM and then a more conspicuous sign stating NO ADMITTANCE. Lee didn't slow down.

He passed through the doors, and to his surprise, he was met by still another set of double doors. This time a white-clad orderly and a formidable-looking nurse attempted to stop him. They shouted, "You may not enter the operating room. You are not prepped for surgery! Besides, we have been scrubbed and ready to begin for ten minutes."

Lee stated firmly, "My wife is about to have a major cancer operation and I haven't seen her or been with her." Pushing his way through the doors, he was confronted by two women wearing white. "*You may not go any further!*" they warned, but they were careful not to touch him.

Lee insisted, "I must see my wife. If I can't come in, you can wheel her out!"

One of the nurses conceded. "Just a second. Step back outside a minute and I'll see what I can do."

He stepped back and waited. Within a moment she reappeared with a cart and I was on it!

"I'll give you a few minutes. We're not supposed to do this. The doctor was ready to begin."

Then followed the ten tender moments I've already reported. They passed much too quickly.

A nurse was approaching Lee and me in the crowded corridor. I looked up and inquired, "How do you make each one of your eyelashes the same distance from the other?"

The perfectly eyelashed figure in white smiled and began moving my cart back through the two sets of double doors. I didn't care. I was in a state of euphoria. "Take it off," I imagined myself saying, "and don't bother with the anesthetic . . ."

7

Surgery

I was in surgery two hours and ten minutes. During the modified radical mastectomy, Dr. Allen removed all tissues of the right breast and the axillary lymph nodes. The pectoral muscles were kept intact.

Though a friend offered to come to the hospital to be with him, Lee chose to be alone during this time. Steve, our sensitive and tender-hearted college-age son, joined him about five-thirty. At seven o'clock, Dr. Allen called Lee to say that he had removed the breast and there were no complications. He had just seen me in the recovery room; I was fine, very strong, doing beautifully.

There in the lobby, Steve and Lee bowed their heads and prayed together. Specifically they prayed that there would be little or no pain, and if there was discomfort, that I would be capable of bearing it.

At nine o'clock the recovery room called to say that they were taking me to my room and Lee and Steve could come up in fifteen minutes. When they arrived I was just being wheeled down the hall, still unconscious.

"Your hair was pulled back off your face, and you were pale," Lee related. He and Steve stood together side by side next to my bed. Lee kissed my forehead and moistened my brow with a cool cloth. Steve, whose nature is to be silent when he is hurting, remained quiet.

The color was returning to my face.

When I regained consciousness, I remember seeing two look-alike faces gazing down at me with a great deal of compassion. When they came into focus I noticed that one had blue eyes and that the other's were dark.

"How do you feel?" Lee asked.

"Fine," I answered.

"Steve was fantastic—very quiet," Lee said. "Do you have any pain?"

"No, I feel wonderful." And I felt loved. I noticed that an I.V. was attached to my left arm.

"I don't even feel nauseated," I added, attempting a smile.

Sleep was willing me to return to her, which I did, and continued to do, soundly, through the night.

8

First Steps to Recovery

The day following surgery was bright and sunny. But I had a problem. I was unable to urinate. The nurses had helped me into the bathroom sometime in the night where they had poured water into the sink, pleaded, and persuaded. Nothing. They repeated the procedure in the morning. Still no results. I tried too hard and my bladder went into spasm. Uncomfortable beyond description, I recall peeking between six white-stockinged legs through the half-opened bathroom door to see Lee, handsome in his brown sport coat, entering my hospital room.

I felt like a failure. Later I learned that this is a common inability of patients following the first night on I.V. feeding.

Reluctantly, the three nurses helped me back to bed. Lee and I hugged hard. A moment later our pastor arrived. He inquired kindly how I felt. Since he is a casual, nonpretentious type, I told him that I felt great, but that I had this one problem that was making me very uncomfortable.

The traces of a smile hovered around his mouth. "Oh, well, perhaps I'd better not go ahead with the Scripture portion I have selected to read."

I was curious. "Why? What does it say?"

With a full smile on his face he read, "And the Lord will never let me go."

After more Scripture and prayer he left.

My next visitor was Dr. Baker. I got an idea. "Have you ever hypnotized a person's bladder?" I queried. By this time I was experiencing severe pressure and discomfort.

Dr. Baker was again ready to help. I noticed that our audience was larger this time. Nurses appeared from nowhere. Lee and the women in white stood against the wall at the foot of my bed looking both amused and fascinated by this unusual request.

I had confidence that the hypnosis would again be effective and slipped into the hypnotic state easily. Soon I heard the quiet command, "When I tell you, your bladder will completely relax and you will be able to release your urine without effort."

Sure enough, almost immediately after I woke up I was able to accompany a nurse to the bathroom where I experienced relief.

I drifted into a comfortable sleep and awakened to discover the college's chaplain standing in the entrance of my room. He told me of the many on campus who were concerned and praying. It was a pleasant, encouraging visit.

Lee came and shared two special letters of love with me.

Then one of my tennis friends arrived. With her blond hair drawn back from her fine-featured face, she resembled a blue and gold Scandinavian angel. Bunny, part-time nurse at the hospital, told me that she would like to volunteer to be with me during my recuperation. Then she handed me a wrapped package. I opened it to discover a little book titled *Streams in the Desert*. I hadn't seen a copy of it for more than twenty-five years, but I well remembered its being in my mother's hands almost daily when I was growing up. She, along with two million others, turned to it for confidence and assurance in God's message for the day.

It was a timely gift, and I told Bunny so. She suggested we share the selection for that day, February 2. I drank it in thirstily as she read:

February 2

"In the shadow of his hand hath he hid me, and made me a polished shaft; in his quiver hath he hid me" (Isa. 49:2).

But fear not! It is the shadow of God's hand. He is leading thee. There are lessons that can be learned only there.

He is keeping thee close till the moment comes when He can send thee most swiftly and surely on some errand in which He will be glorified.

I marveled at the appropriateness of the words. Together, we looked back at the reading for Monday, the day I received that unexplainable quiet immediately before receiving the news of my malignancy, and then again after arriving at the hospital.

Somehow, I was not surprised to read:

January 31

"He giveth quietness" (Job 34:29).

Quietness amid the dash of the storm. We sail the lake with Him still. Suddenly a great storm sweeps down. Earth and hell seem arrayed against us, and each billow threatens to overwhelm. Then He arises from His sleep, and rebukes the winds and the waves. His voice is heard above the scream of the wind in the cordage and the conflict of the billows, "Peace, be still!" *And there is instantly a great calm.*

He draws nigh, and whispers the assurance of His presence. Thus an infinite calm comes to keep our heart and mind.

By then we couldn't resist looking at the reading for the day of surgery:

February 1

"This thing is from me" (1 Kings 12:24).

"Life's disappointments are veiled love's appointments."

Are you in difficult circumstances? This thing is from Me. I am the God of circumstances. Thou camest not to thy place by accident, it is the very place God meant for thee.

The readings moved me to tears. Truly, God did love me and had a purpose and plan for my life. I felt richly reassured of His presence. And I was grateful for caring friends like Bunny who took time from their busy lives to reach out and communicate His love.

9

Concentrating on the Positive

February 3

I awoke feeling frisky. No more I.V. feeding. After devouring scrambled eggs and bacon, I bathed and took time to curl my hair and apply eye makeup. I even curled my eyelashes. This was a sure sign of being on the road to recovery, Dr. Baker told me when he arrived. He had me demonstrate my tennis strokes with my right arm.

"Now let's see your forehand stroke," he instructed, "That's right, take it back. All the way. Wonderful. Now let me see your backhand. Good!" He was immensely pleased with my progress.

Intelligent man. He wanted to see if the hypnosis had worked. It had. No wonder he was pleased. He wasn't half as pleased as I. I was already looking forward to returning to the courts. What really encouraged me was when Dr. Baker suggested that Lee bring my tennis racket to the hospital that afternoon. Using it to practice my strokes would be an ideal way to loosen up my right arm. I was also to begin standing close to the wall, facing it, and run my right arm up the wall as far as I could.

I tried this. It became more uncomfortable the higher the fingers climbed towards the ceiling. I preferred using my tennis racket. It felt like a familiar friend helping me shorten

50

the distance between me and the active world to which I was accustomed. I wondered whether my serve would be affected.

I had the answer the next day. Lee and I were taking a walk down the long hall when we passed an orthopedic surgeon who specializes in tennis injuries. I recognized him from a mixed doubles tennis tournament we had participated in the previous fall. He must have recognized me for he commented, "Your serve will be better than ever." This sounded marvelous. My serve could stand a lot of improvement. It was the weakest part of my game.

Dr. Allen stopped by for a checkup and a chat. He said he hadn't seen any of his mastectomy patients recover faster. We again discussed the possibility of augmentation. This is an increasingly popular operation for breast reconstruction after the removal of a breast.

The greatest source of discomfort to me while in the hospital was having to wear a contraption called a hemovac. It consisted of a plastic sac for collecting the unpleasant-looking yellowish fluid from my side and two long drain tubes which connected the sac with the area of the incision. Several times each day a nurse would drain the fluid from the sac, measure it, and note the amount on a pad. The hemovac was clumsy and sometimes painful. Because my right breast had been removed, I slept on my left side. The long tubes that originated from the wound became tangled between my legs as I moved in the night. Often when I turned, I would forget what I was wearing and the tubes would pull.

To conceal this unsightly appendage I placed the plastic bag in my knitting basket which was on the floor by my bed. When I got out of bed or walked down the hall, I carried the plactic bag in my hand. While chatting with friends, I would slip it out of sight into the folds of my robe. It was repulsive to look at, and I remember feeling self-conscious with visitors as I tried to give them my complete attention and at the same time hide the hemovac.

I do not recall taking any medication, although some may have been given right at the first. I felt that it was a generous gift from God that I wasn't experiencing any pain. The reading I did and my inquiries of other mastectomy patients indicated that absence of pain was unusual. I continued to simply place my total trust in God to see me through. I also trusted in Dr. Allen and Dr. Baker and maintained an attitude of expectancy and optimism.

Someone has said that 10 percent of recovery is from medicine and prescribed treatment and up to 90 percent is in the patient's mental attitude. Perhaps that is true. I also believe that hypnotism was a highly effective factor in my rapid, radical recovery. If any of you who are reading this story are facing surgery now or in the future, or have someone close to you who may be, I strongly urge you to try the kinds of things that were so helpful to me. Avail yourself of the support God stands ready to give when you call upon Him. Try to maintain a positive attitude. Read your Bible and other devotional material that has been meaningful to you. *It will help.*

At no time before or since that wondrous week in the hospital following my mastectomy have I experienced such an overwhelming awareness of the presence of God. My entire being felt like singing, like dancing, like laughing. At last I knew the meaning of the word *joy.* And there is nothing— nothing—like it. It came from within and it bubbled constantly until it spilled over and lifted the lives of others.

Communicating with God—two-way communication— was the most important thing in the world to me during those days. I don't mean communicating with him on a basis of equality, but on a basis of dependency. I had to talk with Him and He with me, because only He perfectly knew my condition and circumstances and only He could perfectly guide me and supply me with coping power through those days.

My tennis racket was mounted on the wall over my hospital bed. I took it out into the hall regularly and practiced my strokes, concentrating on my backswing. I was determined to loosen up the area under my arm as soon as possible. Simply having my racket there provided a promise of brighter days ahead.

Candy's favorite coach had sent a tennis ball to the hospital on which he had printed in large red letters, MRS. CLAUSEN, GET WELL SOON, adding his name. I took this tennis ball out into the hall and tossed it against the wall over and over, each time attempting to increase my flexibility and the number of consecutive catches. It did, and also made me feel good that I was doing something to hasten me towards a full recovery. Soon I completed 49 catches out of 50 tosses. Fortunately, my room was at the end of the hall and I wasn't blocking traffic. On one of these occasions a nurse paused to watch, and then commented, "Gee, I can't throw the ball that consistently myself and I haven't had any surgery!"

I firmly believe that anything you can do to make yourself feel better about yourself and your circumstances will improve your mental attitude. The day after surgery I asked one of the nurses if there was any way she could wash my hair for me. I was wearing it shoulder length then, and it felt and looked yucky. Sure enough, that evening, when things had quieted down on our floor, she supplied a basin and gave me a gentle shampoo.

Since I was not on a strict schedule, I enjoyed taking time with my appearance. Each morning before breakfast I washed, applied fresh makeup, turned under the ends of my hair with a curling wand, and put on my favorite robe, a long green and white gingham check trimmed in ruffles and lace. It made me feel feminine to wear it, and right then, more than any other time in my life, I wanted to feel attractive. Since I was heavily bandaged, I had no visible reminder that one side of my chest was flat.

In his book *Pulling Your Own Strings*, Dr. Wayne W. Dyer tells us that there are always options. In every situation in life, we can choose how we are going to deal with it and how we are going to feel about it. Wherever we are, whatever the circumstances, we can make the situation into a learning or growing experience. Whether this is in a hospital bed, a routine job, in New York City or Wide-Spot-in-the-Road, Missouri—the setting is irrelevant. We can be alive enough to get something out of the experience. He says further that our capacity to be creatively alive in nearly all our situations will depend in large part upon the kind of attitude we choose. The most crucial test of attitude development will be in the face of adversity, rather than while things are running smoothly.

I also knew it was important to feel good about one's inner self. By staying in tune with God and keeping in open communication with Him, I experienced a serenity of spirit. I rediscovered the truth of the teaching, "to the extent that you center your life on God, you will experience His peace." Being confined to a hospital room was for me an ideal time to meditate, to read spiritually inspiring books, (even though I could concentrate on the printed page for only short periods of time) to listen to sacred music on my radio, and to pray.

More than ever I needed His peace. I sought it; I received it. A Bible verse learned in my youth was confirmed in a new way: "And when you draw close to God, God will draw close to you" (James 4:8).

But perhaps the most significant thing that happened to me while I was in the hospital was a discovery that had to do with the other cancer in my life—the one that had invaded my marriage.

In my journal entry for this day I wrote: "Lee is supportive and sexy. I think I'm beginning to love him again. Something magical is happening. God is releasing love held in reserve—each for the other. It is flowing freely together with His love. He is my miracle God. I am in adventure with Him."

10

Plastic Pretenders

The tenderness now growing between Lee and me was in sharp contrast to the feelings we had let develop toward each other over most of the years of our marriage. The malignancy reached unbearable proportions one Sunday in the fall of 1974. . . .

Our family had just returned from church, which we attended every Sunday morning. From all outward appearances we were an ideal American family enjoying life in an upper middle-class, white, suburban area. Mother and Daddy, flanked by two boys and two girls each glowing with good health and good looks, occupied the same pew in the front row on the left side of the sanctuary. When others asked how I was, I smiled and said fine and moved easily into small talk about our latest social event or the rising prices in the grocery store. Arriving home, I fled to the bathroom.

I let the tears flow; they poured down my face streaking the makeup I had carefully applied two hours earlier. Who cared? The "Happy Homemaker" role was over for the day. A total sense of hopelessness and aloneness overcame me, and my sobs grew louder as I remembered the scalding argument Lee and I had had in the car on the way home. Fortunately, the children were in their own car. Bitterness had surfaced and angry words were exchanged. *When was it*

going to end? How many years could one continue under
such separateness without cracking under the terrible tension? My head ached, my heart ached, and my gut ached.
However, I had to get hold of myself, douse my swollen red
eyes with cold water and go prepare dinner—*and act as
though nothing was wrong.* I wondered whether we were
fooling the children. *I am sick of this pretending,* I wept bit-
terly. I am tired of forcing pleasant table conversation when
my heart is breaking. I wanted to run, disappear, *anything*
to escape the hostile feeling of resentment I felt towards
Lee. Prayer, determination, marriage counselors, searching
in books, vacations—*nothing* had helped for any sustained
period of time.

What people in that church on this morning and most of
the others in our lives didn't know was that Lee and I were
plastic pretenders, putting on a front. Our hearts were
breaking and we didn't know how to heal the deep-seated
hurts. Some fifteen years earlier we began to lose that special something that characterized a close, companionable
marriage. But what had gone wrong? We had met at a Christian college, dated for four years, enough time to discover
new qualities in each other and to find that we shared many
of the same interests. We didn't get married until we had
finished college. Our first several years had had their share
of friction but also their share of good feelings and meaningful memories.

And then something happened. It was as though a malignancy invaded the relationship and we each turned to other
interests. I became absorbed in discovering a sense of personal identity, being a competent mother, pouring affection
on my friends, and reading voraciously. I wanted to stretch
my mind, to discuss ideas, and in these pursuits my husband
was no longer my number one priority.

Lee was—and is—a charmer. He exudes male mag-
netism. He was flattered by feminine attention and is constantly showered with it. The time came when I was no

longer the focus of his affections. I felt threatened by attractive women who teased and flirted with Lee. Resentment and jealousy seethed and simmered on the back burner and often boiled over. Frequently we arrived home from parties in screaming silence, and it was simply a matter of moments before the accusations began and the volcano erupted.

As the distance between us widened, I began to think that I didn't love the man I had married and, what's more, I didn't like him either. We tried everything, but the enormous sense of separateness continued. Respect had been replaced with suspicion.

For twelve years we had a summer cottage in the Wisconsin Northwoods. As soon as school was out in the spring, I left with the children to spend the summer, while Lee, busy building his own nursery business, remained in the Chicago suburbs. When he joined us for long weekends, he was looking forward to spending quiet time with the children and me. Meanwhile, during the week, I had devoured thought-provoking books, done things constantly with the children, and couldn't understand why Lee didn't want to discuss the latest book I was reading or go with friends to a favorite restaurant. Our needs, because of our different lifestyles, were in opposite veins. Instead of relationship-building vacations, weekends became "Why can't you understand *me*?" arguments. When Lee left early Monday mornings to return to the city, instead of a warm kiss our goodbye most times consisted of a squeal of tires and angry threats.

We continued in our separate worlds, losing ourselves in everything and anything but each other. Though each made enormous efforts to reach out and rediscover the spark that we had lost, we were able to rekindle a relatedness for only limited lengths of time. Always, always, for the sake of the children, we kept up appearances, confining our arguing as much as possible to the car or going for long walks to let out our feelings.

And then in the summer of 1974 Lee accompanied a large

group of teenagers from our church to Jamaica where they were responsible for organizing and teaching a Bible school. Lee did a lot of the preaching, and during those two weeks he witnessed the power and the love of God as he never before had. When he returned, he didn't resemble the same man who had kissed me goodbye at the airport. He was changed, a brand-new person, humbly made alive to his God and to His power and presence. Lee had been encouraged too by the effect the mission project had had on our son, Steve, who also renewed his Christian commitment.

As Lee made a total about-face, once again I became the target of his affections. He committed himself with an abundance of desire to being a loving and faithful husband. Though I noticed a new tenderness and a more positive attitude, I could not forgive him for the terrible turmoil that had built up inside of me and I was unable to respond to the changes in him. The scars went too deep. Lee's Jamaica spiritual experience was like a Band-Aid on a cancer and I needed much more.

On that unbearable Sunday late in autumn, 1974, I was struggling for any small source of hope in order to survive through the day. Suddenly I recalled the name of a minister given to me by a friend. I decided to go see him that very afternoon. I blotted my tear-streaked eyes, blew my nose, and went downstairs to serve dinner.

I left as soon as the dishes were cleared and loaded into the dishwasher. Rev. Winter asked me many questions, listening carefully as I supplied a history of our marriage beginning with the day we exchanged vows. While I was talking, I noticed that he would lean his head back with his eyes closed, as if he were wired into another source from which he was receiving messages.

After I had brought him up to date, he said that he would like to place his hands on my head and pray, silently at first, and then aloud. He asked that I repeat a prayer after him. As I complied, I wept copiously.

And then something significant took place. Rev. Winter was given a prophecy which he pronounced aloud in slow, distinct phrases. It was utterly beautiful, phrased in the old English language of the Scriptures. It flowed forth—full of hope and promise. It went something like this: "My daughter, I love you very much. Continue to be faithful, keep My commandments, obey My precepts, and someday I will bless you richly, you and your household. Cling to Me and in time you will be rewarded." His hands were still on my head and I knew a sense of profound peace. There it was, the hope I so desperately craved. I was lightened, lifted, and filled with a sense of wonder. I drove home in a state of reverent awe combined with a deep-centered quiet. Also, a renewed determination to be a loving, obedient and faithful wife.

The next day I phoned Rev. Winter and asked him whether he could give me a copy of the prophecy. He said that he didn't know what he had said. He had merely been a medium of a message that he had been given from God for me. He said that he could set aside a designated period of time for prayer and meditation in order to recapture it, but I said no, it was enough to be reminded that God had a brighter future ahead for our marriage.

11

Mission in Jamaica—Lee's Story

Something happened in Jamaica that I had never experienced before. In April of 1974 I made a significant decision to make my life totally different from what it had been for the past ten years. I needed to know for myself whether there was a Power outside of me.

I had been playing the surface rules of the Christian life for ten years—teaching Sunday School, being sensitive to other people's spiritual needs, attending church faithfully, and reading the Bible—and yet I wasn't experiencing what was promised from the pulpit. I asked myself over and over, "What is the missing ingredient? What is wrong? What do I have to do to make my marriage and Christian faith work?"

I was tired of trying to put into practice the formulas that guaranteed a successful marriage. I had been following these suggestions for years, and Janie and I continued to be miles apart. It seemed that whenever a point of crisis or a difference of opinion occurred in our relationship, if I wasn't willing to give or change, the situation erupted into an explosion. At this time I was a 44-year-old, mature, educated, experienced-in-life father and husband, and I felt that I was exhausting my ability to change, to love, and to adjust to the personality changes that were being requested of me. I was ready to stop trying altogether or else to find *something* or *someone* who could help us.

I can identify with the individual who has reached the
end of his struggles with his marriage commitment or the
end of his commitment to his God. I believe that it is
important that we are aware that we may reach the point in
life when we are ready to "toss in the towel" on life's
commitments. I did.

The increasing number of broken marriages and fouled-up
Christian lives proves that people need trained help, that
they need to be listened to, but most of all that they need
someone *who cares for them enough* with whom they can
be totally honest and vulnerable—someone who can listen
without responding in condemnation or castigation. The
Christian community today is ineffective because people like
myself are struggling to play the game of Happy Christian
Couple. I couldn't risk allowing anyone to know where I
really was or where our marriage really was. How many
times I was told, "Be grateful for what you have. There are
so many couples who are worse off than you are." What
ineffective counseling that is!

Should not the Christian community be a hospital—a
welcome place for people with sick marriages—defeated
lives—pain-filled problems? My experience has been that it
is the last place to bring one's doubts, mistakes, and
weaknesses.

I often think of the encounter we had with a so-called
marriage counselor. We spent the best part of a week in
deep, hurting sessions, arguing, pulling apart years of
agony, etc., with the promise, "It will be worth it. You two
will work it out and will be able to get along the way you
are longing to." When the week ended, this man with all
the answers was late getting home to his wife with whom
we had a tentative date to meet and go out for dinner. She
tore into her husband in such a way that we were not
invited into the house or introduced to her. We drove him
to the station. She was so angry with him (and probably
us!) that she was unable to be socially polite. Was *I*

discouraged? You bet I was! The expert with all the answers was failing miserably in his own home!

This was my mental and spiritual condition as I entered the serious phase of my Jamaican experience.

Several months earlier I had begun to attend a weekly session that was preparing thirty-five high school kids to go to Jamaica on a short-term mission project. The kids and their leaders were learning to teach Jamaican young people the Bible.

During these months I decided that *things had to change*. For a few months things were better in our home. Then a slight crisis occurred, and I caught some sort of a virus and ended up in the hospital. By this time I hated hospitals. For the first few days all I could think was . . . here it goes again . . . a decision to try one more time and something inevitably goes wrong. It seemed to be the same tape playing over and over. Maybe we needed a whole new tape.

I arrived home from the hospital very discouraged with my doctor's orders to remain quiet for three weeks! At the end of this time the group was scheduled to leave for Jamaica. Should I plan to go with them? I wanted to; Janie didn't want me to. Another difference of opinion. Something inside me kept encouraging me to go. Would Janie be mad? Could I afford still more time off work? After all, I had missed four weeks already. I had to make up my mind.

"I'll go. I need the opportunity to share myself and my feelings," I said to myself. "Perhaps something will happen in Jamaica that will help me. . . ."

I went. *It turned out to be one of the most important decisions of my life.*

Within the first hour after our arrival in Jamaica, things began to happen. I became aware of some sort of spirit. People that I had known for years were acting and reacting to one another differently. We were being transported thirty-five miles on a sugar cane truck. Steve, our 18-year-old son, and I were standing together on the front of the truck viewing the Jamaican hillsides and the Jamaican people for the first time. Our eyes met and we shared a mutual good feeling, something that was to occur many more times as the weeks progressed. (As I look back now, I believe that this was the beginning of my experiencing true Christian love. What a difference from anything I had known before!)

The week and a half in Jamaica were busy, busy days. They began with cleaning a school so we had a place to live and sleep, repairing toilets and water systems, and finding something to sleep on so that we could get off the concrete floor. We learned to help cook, arrange meetings and classes and most of all, reach out and love Jamaican kids. The 200 kids we expected turned into 600 and we had our hands full. I was called upon to lead meetings, explain over and over how God loves, cares, and wants each of His creatures to be completely content with himself, and where he belonged in this life.

But, what I thought was to happen to the Jamaican kids and to their parents *was happening to me. Life began to take on new meaning.* I couldn't wait for the sun to come up in the morning so I could get out of bed. Sharing life with people was fantastic. When the day ended and darkness came, I crawled into my bedroll and stared out at the Jamaican sky. Tears welled in my eyes and my every emotion was touched. That "something" or "someone" was really happening in my life. *The feeling of love I had longed for was finally there!* Never had the day sky been so blue, the nights so bright—but best of all was the inner security of knowing that I was on the right track at last. God was there, He did care for me, and the spirit to love, feel, and care for other people was there. What a terrific sensation *that* is.

Jamaica ended. I cried when I left. I didn't want to leave the place that had become so precious to me. My dear son

Steve and I were able to hold each other, talk with each other in depth, pray together, and shed tears together.

Well, half of the struggle was over. God and I were truly on speaking and listening terms. Now, what about Janie? Could I ever explain it all to her? Could she understand? Was it too late for this marriage to be happy again? The flight home from Jamaica was one I'll never forget!

The ecstasy and anticipation of acceptance and love, or the agony of being rejected, doubted, and questioned—which was it to be?

12

The High Price of Stress

My parents were not demonstrative; they rarely hugged or kissed us, their children. I never remember being told "I love you." Although they loved us, I did not *feel* loved. This contributed to my inability to express love and affection in marriage.

The importance of being obedient to authority was stressed in my childhood, of toeing the mark. Meeting the needs of his congregation was more of a priority for Daddy than spending time with his children. Mother was concerned with the appearance of the manse—the minister's home—and whether we were being shining examples. Occasionally we were invited, one at a time, to accompany Daddy in the car on an errand, but I felt uncomfortable, awkward, and alone with him.

"What can I say that would attract his attention to *me?*" I wondered. "Why doesn't he talk to me? If only he would reach out and give me a hug or let me know that he likes me or approves of me, it might make that lonely place inside of me go away." I was to spend a large portion of my life trying to capture my father's attention, approval, and affection.

For years I was insecure and lacked a sense of personal worth. I felt that I needed to *do* certain things in order to earn approval. It didn't occur to me that *who I was* was more important that *what I did*. I felt that my worth to my parents lay not in myself, but in something else—in my appearance, my actions, in getting good grades, and in being and doing what was expected of me.

My dad, possessing a magnetic personality and enormous charm, had a large number of female admirers. He was a popular, well-liked pastor with a large capacity to listen to the problems of his congregation. Mother was threatened by all this attention, and we overheard arguments that indicated her intense jealousy.

Lee was the only boy in a family of three sisters. From his earliest days he has been fawned over by females. Throughout our marriage his athletic good looks, teasing humor, and outgoing personality have attracted the attention of the opposite sex. He, like my father, was accustomed to an abundance of attention and affirmation. Though most of these were harmless flirtations, I found myself extremely jealous, as my mother had been. I simply could not adjust to Lee's ability to make other women feel special.

I began seeking to establish my own identity, to be someone more than just "Lee's wife" and the children's mother. I read everything I could get my hands on about self-awareness. I learned terms like transactional analysis, parent-effectiveness, self-actualization. To stretch my mind I read C. S. Lewis, Paul Tournier, Erich Fromm, Dietrich Bonhoeffer, and Sam Shoemaker. I devoured Reuel L. Howe, Keith Miller, and Bruce Larson. The fact was that I was no longer satisfied with myself as I was or with my husband as he was.

In my search for that extradimensional person inside me, I came across a magazine article which confirmed that there were other women besides me who needed a more accepting, positive attitude towards themselves. The article grabbed my attention for several other reasons. When Lee arrived at the cottage that weekend I was anxious to share it with him. I waited for just the right moment and then asked him to read it. His reaction was negative. "Why can't you just be happy, Janie? You have so much for which to be thankful!" (I was sick of hearing him say this over and over like a broken record.) After that, I felt even lonelier and more aware of our inability to meet one another's needs.

Unable to stimulate Lee's interest in these intellectual pursuits, I began to replace him with books, thoughts, ideas, the children, tennis, friends, family—anything. And he replaced me. Heartbreaking, painful years followed. It seemed so simple—and yet so difficult. Here we were—two people who had fallen in love, married, had four beautiful, healthy children, and yet each was desperately lonely, desperately needing love. We had reached a stalemate.

We went to a series of marriage counselors. I read books on improving the marriage relationship, collected articles on "Ways to Be a Good Wife," studied sex manuals, and prayed to be able to meet Lee's needs. But things grew worse. The gap became a chasm. Wounds occurred. Threats. Shouting sessions. Pleadings. Broken promises.

One day I discovered the wonderful truth that God loved me exactly as I was—with all of my faults. There is a divine order, Pete Gillquist told me in his book *Love Is Now:* "Jesus loves me first, I love myself because He loves me. Now that I love myself, I am free to love others." Loving ourselves means accepting our weaknesses as well as our strengths. God loves me unconditionally *as I am*. He loves others *as they are*. God made us as we are for a reason. Concentrate on God's love, Mr. Gillquist advised. He has confidence in us—His unique creation.

He went on to say that we should trust His Spirit to lead us into a new adventure with Him. His book freed me from misconceptions I had possessed for years. I thought about this and prayed for it to happen to me. A new adventure. . .

Meanwhile, Lee had slipped into some self-depreciating patterns. He was not pleased with his behavior. Afflicted by a sense of personal worthlessness, he hated his own inadequacy and futility. Soon he was hating *himself.* "Why am I doing this?" he asked himself. The tendency was to conclude, "Oh, well, I'm bad already, so I might as well continue." When this anger turned in on himself, he became depressed and despondent. When I questioned how he had been spending his time, and with whom, he became defensive and exploded in fury.

Lee overreacted to my accusations and I withdrew from his overt anger into silence. I saw Lee as weak. My respect for him had vanished. But my negative response to his weakness only contributed to it. My behavior did not invite him to reach out and care for me. I had turned into a suspicious, unforgiving, and jealous woman, and I began to suspect that I no longer loved Lee.

Why didn't we get a divorce?

I'm not sure. Perhaps it was because my conservative minister father had trained us to believe that divorce is a sin in the sight of God. I had the fear of God in me. My behavior was an alarming carbon copy of my mother's reactions to the female adulation her husband had received.

Second, it would be admitting failure, and I was never a quitter.

Third, whenever we discussed a possible divorce or separation, neither of us could consider parting with the children. I recall echoes of his blistering pronouncement, "You leave, if you don't like it, and I'll stay with the children." How could I face life without *them?*

Most important of all, *I* would not approve of divorce. It appeared as though something drastic would have to happen to change things.

"Oh God, where are You?" I agonized. "Why don't You answer my prayers? Are You there? I am desperate. Please change our marriage. Please change Lee. Please change me. I am trapped in a tunnel that has no exit. Lee simply doesn't understand me. I have no more strength, no more fight. I am hopelessly alone. I cannot hold myself together. I am being poured out. I am losing, losing. What is there left to do to save our desolate marriage? Please help me make it through this day—through this hour."

This was often my heart's prayer in the 1960's and 1970's. But I don't think I ever stopped believing in the reality of God and constantly pleaded for His strength, His power and His comfort.

It has been generally accepted that emotional stress expresses itself in bodily stress. It has also been suggested that people show only one-tenth of their true, recognized feeling to others, and are themselves consciously aware of only a small part of their own emotions. We hide the bulk of our emotions even from ourselves by the defense mechanism called repression.

In *The Secret of Staying in Love,* John Powell talks about the effects of repressing our emotions. He reports that the non-expression of emotions is very common. And the expression of emotions into the subconscious is even more self-destructive, he says, because repressed emotions do not die. They pervasively influence the whole personality and behavior of the repressor. Repressed fears and angers may be "acted out" physically as insomnia, headaches, or ulcers. Buried emotions are like rejected people; they make us pay a high price for having rejected them. Hell hath no fury like that of a scorned emotion.

Lee paid a high price indeed. Because of a lifestyle that was not consistent with his better judgment and value system, he was living with guilt, and rather than confess the wrong actions, he repressed his guilt feelings. One of the reasons he was afraid to confess his behavior to me or to our minister was because of the probability of rejection.

What resulted was a series of illnesses for Lee, including a severe virus, a hemorrhoidectomy, back problems that demanded traction, a staphylococcal infection, and heart problems. Over a period of ten years he was hospitalized every two years. Four of these five occasions were in February.

Why February? The landscaping business is seasonal. Our income in the winter is based on snow removal and the sale of firewood. February is often the slowest month for work and the time of the year when Lee spends more time at home. Thus he and I were thrust together more than usual in February, with more time to think about our deeply troubled marriage.

At the end of February 1978, Lee entered the hospital for extensive tests on his heart. The results were encouraging. Though he did not require open heart surgery he must carry medication on his person for an artery which occasionally goes into spasm.

How did I handle my stress? Since my teenage years I have played tennis regularly. By pounding the small yellow ball I am able to vent a certain amount of tension and frustration. And one cannot play tennis alone. By being with another human being, usually someone who cares for me, my depression is at least temporarily relieved. However, I remember the familiar body changes when Lee and I were having a particularly severe disagreement. Invariably, I would shiver with cold and more than once developed diarrhea.

An article that appeared in *Lady's Circle* in February 1980 focused on stress and its relation to cancer. It reported recent studies showing that stress could seriously inhibit the body's immune system, which ordinarily prevents the survival of abnormal or harmful cells. Dr. Paul J. Rosch, then vice president of the New York State Society for Internal Medicine, pointed out that the incidence of cancer of the breast and uterus is much higher among widows than among married women in the same age group. He also cited research findings that showed tumor development in animals to be greatly increased under stressful conditions, and significantly reduced when the animals were insulated against stress.

Dr. Rosch emphasized the importance of holding a strong

belief in one's ability to cope and to maintain good health. In his opinion, a positive attitude is a strong factor in remissions among some cancer patients, and with fantastic "cures" among so-called faith healers.

Undoubtedly, one's emotional, psychological and spiritual health is directly related to our physical health.

I believe that there are several varieties of wife-failure. One of these is the inability to create a positive, mental climate in the home. I was unable to do this. I needed to learn the art of tactfulness. Above all, I needed to cultivate the habit of acceptance; to love my husband as he truly *was*. That's what mature love does.

The secret of staying in love is communication. Indeed, our greatest gift to each other is a gift of self through the honest sharing of feelings and emotions. A growing relationship requires commitment to that open and genuine expression which can occur only in a climate of love, and, I failed to provide a climate of love in our home. It's been said the woman is the barometer of the emotional climate of the home. In my search for self-identity I neglected Lee's psychological and emotional needs. His physical desires didn't fluctuate as much as mine. With regard to love-making, I failed to communicate my highs, lows, and in-betweens, and Lee had to guess them from my moods and actions. Some weren't pleasing. And because I was insensitive to his physical needs, my husband went elsewhere for communication and companionship.

Because I did not experience affection as a child I was unable to spontaneously reach out to touch or hug my husband even though I craved to be held and touched. The dilemma went unresolved because each of us wanted the other to reach out first.

I used to hate the passage in the Bible that states that wives are to be submissive to their husbands. The truth is that I needed to change from a naturally domineering woman to a gentle and sensitive one with a meek and quiet spirit. Years later I learned that submission is an attitude of the heart. It's not so much what we do, but the attitude in which we do what is right. Because I did not possess a forgiving spirit, I may have hindered the work of God. Forgiving Lee wouldn't have made his wrong right, but it would have cleared the way for God to work in me.

Lee had already begun to move away from his emotionally dependent position when he returned from Jamaica, a renewed man. And, when he made a transition towards accepting responsibility for his own happiness, it had a liberating effect on me. I responded positively to this new attitude. He gradually found himself less resentful, freed from my impossible, heartbreaking expectations. He no longer felt abused when he didn't get the reactions he wanted.

While in Jamaica, Lee had received a total acceptance of the unconditional love of God. He had come to the end of himself, asked for forgiveness, and asked God to make him a brand new person. God, in turn, had provided Lee with an overwhelming sense of His power and presence. The change in him was soon visible. His attitude towards God, himself, and me had changed for the better. The deep love of the team who went along with him to sing and teach as well as the warm acceptance of the Jamaicans had profoundly affected him. He returned to his family with a determination to live out this love in his relationships with the significant people in his life, beginning with me.

A tangible result of the changed Lee was his decision to discontinue self-depreciating personal habits. He began by breaking off a significant, unsanctioned relationship that didn't contribute to his self-respect. He began to assume responsibility for his former actions. Each week for one year he met with three deacons. Lee endeavored to become a loving, responsible, and faithful husband.

During those years before Lee's personal encounter with God in Jamaica, it is my opinion that he depended on me for a sense of well-being. He expected to live through me rather than with me as a partner. A woman and man can support each other to some extent in marriage. But each also needs to take a central role in the responsibility for self. I don't think that previously Lee knew much about the responsibility he must take for his own satisfaction, in marriage and in life. Lee returned to me from Jamaica well on the road to self-respect and wholeness. With God's help he was willing to rebuild a permanent, dependable, supporting, companionable marriage partnership which nonetheless didn't have to be the be-all and end-all of existence.

One September day shortly after Lee's return from Jamaica, I received a devastating phone call. It came from a really dear friend of mine and it shattered my world. She revealed long-term secrets—names, places, dates—that left me feeling utterly betrayed. Our marriage came close to dissolving when all the long-suppressed problems finally surfaced as a result of this phone conversation.

Unrecognized and unexamined anxiety festers until it erupts. Sometimes it is difficult to identify the anxiety unless it emerges by accident. The September phone call was a catalyst that enabled Lee and me to identify the anxiety and friction that had festered so long. What followed was a process of self-examination which eventually resulted in the rekindling of affection.

After my mastectomy, with its countless demonstrations of Lee's caring, I noticed that the two of us were developing a new, if guarded, interest in each other. Although we were anxious about our present exposed relationship, there were signs of renewed interest. Very slowly we were able to talk about specific items that had always caused conflict and pain in the past. It is difficult not to respond to love. Although my emotional pain was deep and I was wrestling to forgive and forget, I was gradually succumbing to Lee's demonstrations of love.

As on the four occasions when I was hospitalized for the children's births, Lee was tender and attentive during visiting hours. His unusually sensitive nature communicated both sympathy and strength. He exuded a quality of comfort in a crisis. I still struggle with tears remembering the look on his face when I regained consciousness after the operation. The entire episode provided an opportunity for me to be reminded of my husband's considerate, comforting bedside manner. His attitude told me, "Everything's going to be all right." His warm, teasing humor was always welcome and kept me from taking myself too seriously.

13

Node News

My roommate, Donna, and I were exhausted. She had en-
dured three hours of disc surgery and it had been a long,
long night. Through most of it the nurses had rolled her from
side to side, as though she were a log. A young woman had
screamed hysterically that the nurses had taken her baby.
(She had been moved to our floor from the maternity floor.)
Hospitals are not private places. We agreed to notify the
switchboard that we would take no incoming calls. We then
shut off the TV, closed the door, and prepared to indulge in
a nap.

No sooner had I snuggled beneath the sheets when the
door moved slowly open and Bobbie and Shari, two tennis
friends, stole into the room. I rebelled within. I was so tired.
And then I thought, they left their nice warm homes, or
perhaps the tennis club, to drive out here and see me. The
least I can do is sit up, look alive, and tune in to them. Shari
had made me a handsome necklace out of genuine turquoise
stones. Bobbie had brought me a unique gift. It was a collection of flip cards mounted on a small stand. There was an individual quote for each day of the year. By flipping the card
over at the beginning of the day, our family is fed spiritual
food as well as physical food for breakfast. Before long we
were caught up in lively girl talk. Bobbie told me that her

family also had Dr. Allen and Dr. Baker, too. She was particularly interested in hearing about hypnotism.

A faint, but indistinct buzz could be heard coming from my phone. I ignored it. Again. There must be some mistake. I had called the switchboard to remind them we had requested no calls.

More chatter.

And another buzz.

My curiosity caused me to pick up the receiver. A male voice asked, "Janie, do you want *soup* or *news?*"

I recognized Dr. Allen's voice.

"I'll take the news!" I was shouting.

"The lab report just arrived. All your lymph nodes were negative! I wanted to call you before my next surgery."

I whispered my "thank you" and sobbed uncontrollably. The girls, both with tears in their eyes, left quietly.

I was in a profound state of gratitude for the good news when a nurse appeared and handed me a stack of cards and letters. As I opened them one by one, I noticed a similarity. People prayed, not that God would heal Janie Clausen, but that His presence would be real to me; second, that He would be my source of strength; and third, that through my experience, He would be lifted up—that others would be drawn to Him, the Source of my peace. Looking back, I can vouch that those prayers were realized.

Inevitably, tears welled up as the many kind, affirming words ministered to my spirit.

From a friend—

In my years of knowing you well, I always viewed you as being a very competitive, strong-of-mind-and-soul kind of person who hardly knew the meaning of the word "lose" in *any* area of life! I know now that God will work through these strengths in your personality to bring you through *this* crisis a "winner"!

In all sincerity,
Jan

From a sister—

I think of you constantly these days and pray that the Lord is giving you the strength only He can give at this time. I love you and want you to know that you mean an awful lot to me. We have shared so many great times together and memories are innumerable. I'm glad we've been able to be together these past few years.

You're special to me, Janie, so please stay at peace. We love you and are praying for you.

Warmly,
Mary

I was still lost in the pages of these loving letters when Dr. Allen walked in.

"Watch out," I announced, "I'm going to hug you until it hurts."

I did. Warm feelings of admiration, appreciation, and affection were communicated in the embrace that followed. He quickly removed the tubes leading from the incision to the hemovac and then said, "Take a look, Janie, at what I've done."

I was reluctant. I wasn't sure that I was ready for this.

"Come on," he insisted. "Take a look. It's beautiful."

I glanced down briefly and saw out of the corner of my eye a long line of black stitches marching across my chest.

"You're healing rapidly. I've been hearing about you. You are so nearly well. You may go home any time now."

It was three days after surgery.

"I don't want to go home. I'm not ready. Too much is happening. I'm tired."

"Listen," he went on, "there's been a serious train accident in Chicago and we might need your bed. The elevated fell off the tracks and the hospital might have to give up some beds. Yours may be needed."

"I'm exhausted emotionally and I need rest." I wasn't ready to face the loving confusion of husband, four active children, a large dog, my mother-in-law, and the telephone.

"I will, if I have to," I heard myself say. He disappeared. I
loved him. I would have done anything for him.

I picked up the phone and notified Lee and the secretary
who was filling in for me in the English Department.

Then, with the radio providing a background of sacred
music and the afternoon sunlight spilling over the snowswept
ground outside, I took my pen in hand to write an important
thank-you note:

Praise you, Jesus.
I am spilling over with a grateful heart.
Sunlight is saturating my soul.
Thank you, God, that:
    —I am free of cancer.
    —that Dr. Baker just took me through a series of exercises
      and stated that my right arm muscle movement is ninety-
      nine percent three days after surgery.
    —I can feel your spirit surrounding me with your quiet
      love.
    —I am flooded with friends.

14

The Power of Love

Saturday morning Dr. Allen dropped in to say that he would be sending me home the next day. He warned me not to push, as I would tire *easily*. He also asked that I call and make an appointment for the following Wednesday at his office.

It surprised me to realize I loved the hospital and was reluctant to leave it. So many good things were happening. Flowers, gifts—each gesture of love made me feel *special* and overwhelmed me with the goodness of people. The constant affection of my doctor, the nurses, and other hospital personnel—I'd be leaving all this.

A visit from an attractive lady named Barbara, from the Reach for Recovery program, lifted my spirits just when they might have sagged in self-pity. Barbara, who had had both of her breasts removed some time earlier, and who loved playing tennis, demonstrated exercises that would help my arm to loosen. She also gave me helpful material from the American Cancer Society: letters for each of our children to help them adjust to their new mother, and a pamphlet for Lee with valuable information for the husband of the mastectomy patient. It was interesting to learn of the variety of prostheses available. Barbara's smile, her neat appearance, and her pleasant personality provided an important source of encouragement.

Another visit that afternoon bolstered me even more. My neighbor, Luci, close friend, horseback-riding companion, and prayer partner, had been out of town when I was suddenly hurled into the hospital for cancer. Just back from her trip, she arrived in my room bringing with her a leather-bound copy of *My Living Counselor*. I cherish this gift from Luci. A talented writer, she ranks high among American poets, and this compilation is her third published book. In it, using the Living Bible paraphrase, she has placed related verses and phrases in creative tension with each other on the page. She suggested we read together for February 5. We started with the morning reading:

> *And the Lord replied, "I myself will go with you and give you success."*
> For the Lord God, the Holy One of Israel, says: . . . in quietness and confidence is your strength. . . .
> Rest in the Lord; wait patiently for him to act. Come to me and I will give you rest—all of you who work so hard beneath a heavy yoke. Wear my yoke . . . and let me teach you; for I am gentle and humble, and you shall find rest for your soul. *Now I can relax. For the Lord has done this wonderful miracle for me . . .*
> You have let me experience the joys of life and the exquisite pleasures of your own eternal presence.

The evening reading was especially meaningful to me:

> I will open up the windows of heaven for you and pour out a blessing so great you won't have enough room to take it in! Try it! Let me prove it to you!

When Luci left, I reflected on this one more unmistakable reminder of God's timing. Each day I had been a living recipient of the outpouring of His blessing. In the normal course of events, people do not communicate their positive feelings in the concrete ways that I'd experienced. But when one is facing a difficult circumstance, those expressions flow forth in torrential quantities. Starved as I had been for affection, the abundance of love that had just been showered upon me was doubly meaningful.

Deliberate efforts to meet human needs, whether by a smile, a letter, a spontaneous hug, a listening ear, the sharing of the right book, a bag of garden tomatoes, or a word of encouragement, do much to lighten another's load. Each expression of love, no matter how insignificant, means a great deal to the one on the receiving end. When people are hurting, defeated, discouraged, or in a crisis, they need to know that we love them. There is no greater gift. It eases the pain, soothes the spirit, and promotes healing and health. I ought to know.

I will never underestimate the power of a loving letter. Words, as well as prayers, can change gray to gold. I hope that I never forget the comfort, the good feelings, or the grateful tears that I experienced while reading the notes and cards I received after my surgery. They serve as a reminder of the importance of telling someone special in my life that he or she matters to me.

15

Welcome Home

Sunday, February 6

Donna and I awoke reluctantly to thermometers and breakfast trays. Mixed emotions about going home were still with me.

I asked Donna whether she would be interested in watching one of my favorite Sunday morning TV programs, "The Hour of Power," a real spirit-builder for me. She said yes and ended up being mesmerized by the hour-long show that emphasized the power of positive thinking in conjunction with the power of God. Donna was hungry to hear more of Him.

Throughout the days we'd been roommates, I had been sharing with her the significance of my faith in God. By this time Donna had become my public relations person, while I became God's public relations person.

On several occasions women would stroll up and down the hall in their bathrobes. Sometimes they would glance into our room. Before you knew it Donna would invite them in. "Come in and meet my roommate, Janie. She's fun and she's religious. Perhaps she can tell you something that will help you." A few would wander in out of curiosity, wanting to know about my electric curling wand which I used each day. One gal was deeply concerned about the outcome of a biopsy on her breast. She and others commented on my smile and sparkle.

"What are you in the hospital for?" one asked. I told her. "How can you possibly be cheerful?" she continued.

I told her and the others about my faith and they listened. It had become more natural to speak of Jesus than not to. The nurses too, were curious about the happy lady in Room 58. They commented on the abundant flower garden and the crowded bulletin board. I shared with them, too, the source of my joy.

The daily reading for February 6 in *My Living Counselor* added emphasis. "The meek will be filled with fresh joy from the Lord."

Since I'd be leaving the hospital in an hour or two and going home to see my family, I took special pains with my appearance. I wanted to do everything I could to get back into the normal routine. I walked down the hall to the large private shower room where I placed my clean clothes on a chair along with shampoo, creme conditioner, and towels. Before stepping into the shower, I walked up to the large mirror and willed myself to pull away the layers of adhesive and gauze. Thinking about it now, I believe this was an important step in my emotional adjustment. I told myself: "My breast has been removed. It is gone—never to be a part of me again. I can become full of self-pity and adopt a why-did-this-happen-to-me attitude. Where will this kind of thinking get me? Nowhere. Wishing won't replace my missing breast. Why not choose to be glad I still have one left—that Dr. Allen got all of the cancer?" This kind of thinking made more sense. It was time to get on with the business of living.

I looked directly into the mirror and counted thirty-one stitches laced with black thread across my chest and around under the armpit to my back.

I noticed something else. Dr. Allen had managed to save extra folds of skin so that augmentation would be possible without skin grafting. This would have to take place sometime after the surgical area had thoroughly healed. Silicone implants were being safely and effectively used for mastectomy patients. It was something I was considering.

The nipple was missing, but the areola, the darkened area that surrounds the nipple, remained. The scar was a horizontal one, perhaps seven inches, running across my chest to my armpit. The skin was only slightly puckered, but there was no hollow—just a narrow line broken by a brownish pink area with enough tissue in which to insert an implant. Dr. Allen was right. It was a fine piece of surgery. No wonder he was so proud.

I shampooed my hair, dressed, and got back into bed for a short rest before applying fresh makeup and curling my hair for the Special Occasion. By the time I had my suitcase packed I was exhausted and decided I needed a nap before the grand exit.

Suddenly Lee, Kim, Candy, Scott, and Elsie burst into the room. The children smiled shyly and we held each other briefly. They had stopped on their way home from church and announced that it had been a "Janie Clausen service." Our pastor had been encouraged by a phone call I had been prompted to make early that morning about my progress. I proudly introduced these very special people to Donna and the members of her family who were visiting her. Then our gang loaded their arms with flowers and plants and said they would be back later for me. They had a few things to do at home and I would have time for lunch and a nap.

Across the hall was an empty room, quiet and inviting. After I finished eating, I slipped into it and grabbed some much-needed rest.

When Lee arrived to take me home I was refreshed, but not emotionally ready to part from the place of my adventure. The leave-taking with Donna was tearful for both of us. Holding her tightly, I kissed her cheek, whispered that Jesus loved her and that I loved her, and promised that we would be in touch.

By the time Lee and I reached the elevator, a great sadness enveloped me, and I could not speak. All the way down the long hall, down five elevator floors, past the checkout desk and on out to the car my lips remained locked.

Finally, when we reached the privacy of our familiar blue station wagon, the dam broke. I wept uncontrollably.

"Why are you crying?" Lee inquired gently.

"I don't know," I murmured, looking out the window as the hospital grew smaller. "I'm so happy to be going home but so afraid the adventure that was taking place in there might be over."

He seemed to understand. He gave me a pair of dark glasses to put on and a well-worn hand to hold.

The house looked the same. The celery shag carpeting, the hand-hewn beams, the rough stone fireplace, the wood-paneled walls seemed to say. "We're glad you're home." We had gathered in our large rustic living room where we looked at the collection of cards and letters, admired the gifts, and belatedly celebrated Steve's twenty-first birthday. Then Steve's girl and I had a long conversation while Lee and the children went to church. There, Lee stood and expressed his gratitude for the neat things that were happening. He returned with a huge pizza and a couple of friends.

It had been a strenuous day. I was content to make myself deliciously comfortable in our king-sized bed while Lee said goodbye to our guests and straightened up the living room.

Suddenly the door to our room opened and Kim appeared, poured into her eighth-grade graduation dress—noticeably braless. She resembled a full-blown princess. In that moment I became sharply aware of my single, slightly sagging breast.

"Mom, can I wear this dress for the concert on the twentieth?" she inquired.

"You'll need a bra." I offered her my "Next-to-Nothing" bra, a Christmas present from Lee two months earlier.

She disappeared to return a moment later. Stretching the

item in her hands, she muttered disgustedly, "It's too small!"
Ouch.

I felt pain. The mental "poor me" variety.

I decided that was enough for my first day home from the hospital, pulled up the covers and turned out the light.

Before going to sleep I wrote the following:

Thank you, Lord, that:
1. Scott told me tonight I was the best mommy in the whole world.
2. Elsie surprised me with new, clean sheets on our muchly missed bed.
3. Candy preferred remaining with me to riding her snowmobile this afternoon.
4. Kim quietly and cheerfully cleaned up the kitchen tonight.
5. Steve's girl told me that she loved me.
6. Lee stood tall and talked about You in church.
7. I was the one to tuck Scott into bed.
8. We are a family reunited.
9. You are going to continue our adventure.

16

Fret Not Thyself

The next day, after hanging up the phone for the fourth time, I got ready for my luncheon date. The day before I left the hospital Katie and Marion had asked me to go with them and one or two others to the Viking, a plush restaurant. I hadn't hesitated. I took my time deciding what to wear, finally settling on camel slacks and a handsome Indian sweater accented with a piece of South American jewelry from sister Mary. With the help of a slightly padded bra and the bandage I appeared to have two breasts. I liked the trimmer image that stared back at me from the bedroom mirror.

And then it hit me. Exactly one week ago today I was also preparing for a luncheon date. At that time I didn't know that I had cancer. And here I was seven days later, the cancer removed, ready to reenter the world of stimulating people and creatively prepared cuisine. It hardly seemed possible.

We giggled and girl-talked our way through Eggs Benedict. I could not keep quiet about God's countless divine appointments. I wanted others to know what the power of God can do to heal cancers of all kinds. It spilled out between bites. They listened intently. One commented with a great deal of solemnity, "I envy you. You don't know how much I envy you."

I was reminded of the reading on the verse-a-day cards from Bobbie.

88 RADICAL RECOVERY

Don't wish yourself in the other fellow's place because he has
a better job, makes more money, lives in a finer house, drives
a better car, dresses better, and has better food than you, unless his inner life is better than yours.

My response was, "You, too, can have the same faith."
As soon as I reached home I disrobed and slid between
the sheets. The glow of being with good friends lingered late
into the afternoon.

My secretarial job had made it impossible for me to be at
home when Scott arrived home from school. Today, of
course, was different. It was an unusually bright, cloud-free
day. Great gobs of sunshine flooded our bedroom with
golden light. Scott's small-boy body invaded it, his fist filled
with second-grade papers.

"Mommy," he announced, sitting down on my bed, "Mrs.
Clark, my teacher, loves you."

"Why does Mrs. Clark love me?"

"Cause," he continued, "I told her you had surgery."

"What did you tell her happened to me?"

"Well, I told her that you had a breast and a limp 'nood'
moved. Right?"

I found his explanation endearing and chose not to correct
his technical description of the surgery. For three days I
searched for the breast that had moved—but without success. I then told Scott that he should place the prefix *re* in
front of the *moved*.

One week after my mastectomy I drove myself to the
clinic for my first post-surgical checkup. Dr. Allen informed
me that everything was healing beautifully. I was lying on
the table when he inserted a giant needle into the area of the
incision and drained a considerable amount of fluid, filling
and emptying the needle twice. The increased pressure
formed by the fluid had caused the stitches to pucker and
turn red. The area had become swollen and uncomfortable
and there was still no relief.

Then Dr. Allen selected a second, still longer needle, and

with me in a sitting position, he removed still more yellowish solution. This time I experienced an enormous release of pressure. Since the nerves had been severed during
surgery, the areas was numb and there was a minimum of
discomfort from the needles.

I mentioned that shooting pains attacked that area at unexpected moments and also that my upper arm was sensitive
and had a sandpapery feeling. He assured me that this was
perfectly normal. Nerves had been severed and raw ends
were healing. I was to make an appointment for the following Wednesday.

The next day Gram, Scott, Kim, Lee and I watched Candy
lead her school basketball team to an overwhelming victory.
She was the superstar, scoring most of the points. We
applauded her noisily. After the game I threw the tennis ball
marked GET WELL across the gym to its sender, her coach. I
loved the creative medium he had used to convey his message. He threw it back, a grin monopolizing his ruddy face.
Once again I tossed it to him shouting, "Read it!" This time
he observed my printed THANKS and came over to talk to me
saying how happy he was to hear the news of my rapid recovery. The school principal added his good wishes. Today,
the unique get-well greeting lettered in red on a tennis ball
still occupies an obvious spot on my desk.

An hour later I drove to the high school to watch Kim sink
baskets for her school team. Occasionally, while captivated
by the team's play, a stabbing pain would snatch my stitches
and I would let go with a loud "Ouch!" I found it increasingly
difficult to smother my ouches. Lee, embarrassed, moved
farther away from me in the bleachers, but I didn't care. The
game was far too exciting. There was Kim, charging towards
the basket with the ball. The ball was tossed in the air and
swish . . . another two points! Only she plunked it through
the hoop of the *opposing* team's basket.

It counted. Her team lost by one point! I was uncomfortable for her. Lee's comment, "It's a growing experience for
her. . . ."

Lee, Bob, Marion, and I donned our party clothes and attended a Valentine's Day dinner, my first appearance at a church function since surgery. I decided on a white ruffled blouse with a scoop neck, a black velveteen vest and a long narrow black slitted skirt. I must admit that I double-checked my chest on the right side before leaving the house. Could anyone else see that it went straight down, instead of rounding out like my left side? I decided that the profusion of ruffles concealed the fact that there was no cleavage on my right side. I had carefully tucked a wad of cotton into my bra. The church was decorated with hearts and flowers, and the people were gracious and loving. I noticed that the men did not treat me differently. I was sensitive to the tenderness in their manner and the wealth of warm feelings, hugs, and happiness that spread around me that evening. I thanked God for the wonder of being alive, surrounded by people who were rejoicing with me in a radical recovery.

After we got home, a friend called and inquired whether I could share my story with her. I explained to her that I was considering a wiser way of relating it. By telling it to one or two at a time (it took close to an hour and a half) I became exhausted. Since Elsie, my mother-in-law, had left, I was handling all of the housework—preparing meals, answering the phone, doing the laundry, etc. It had become both time-consuming and emotionally exhausting to repeat what God had done for me each day. Another friend had offered her family room for me to fill with those who were interested to come and listen over coffee, and I invited the caller to join us then.

The evening ended with still another phone call: to hear a friend's voice say, "It's Valentine's Day, and I'm calling to say that I love you." I melted. I had been warmed one more time by the greatest gift of all.

On Tuesday, February 15, I hardly slept at all after 3:00 A.M. My upper arm was uncomfortable. The stitches were due to come out the next afternoon and I could hardly wait. I got up at 4:30 and did some writing. At 7:00 A.M., when the house had emptied except for Scott, I snuggled back into bed, willing sleep. I had pleaded with Scott, "Please be extra quiet. Mommy didn't sleep last night, and I'm going back to bed now."

One half-hour later I sat upright to the sound of small hands crashing on the piano keys and a blaring TV. I tiptoed downstairs to discover plants and furniture rearranged and an innocent-appearing eight-year-old boy.

I exploded, shouted, scolded, and slammed two doors with such force that I hurt my sensitive right arm.

A short time later I sat down to read the daily reading in my new companion, *Streams in the Desert.*

"Fret not thyself" (Psalm 37:1).

Do not get into a perilous heat about things! Keep cool! Even in a good cause, fretfulness is not a wise help-meet.

After a hand-applied-to-the-bottom talk, Scott was duly sobered and the room returned to order. The blue hairbrush had been neglected far too long.

Later that evening Scott snuggled up to me and whispered, "Mommy, I have a Valentine love message for you." And he handed me an envelope. Inside he had written how much he loved me.

Candy was in her room, uncomfortable with a recently repaired tooth. She was nursing a temporary filling and requested something soft to eat.

"Scott, would you please save Mommy some steps and take Candy a dish of Jell-O?"

His customary answer would be of the negative variety.

This time it went like this: "O.K., Mommy, but only if you will give me a big kiss."

I made a mental note to use the blue hairbrush more often.

February 16

I told my miracle story for the first time to a public gathering. A diversified collection of acquaintances had gathered. Their response alternated between tears and laughter.

I ended my talk with the reading for that day from *Streams in the Desert*:

"Though I have afflicted thee, I will afflict thee no more" (Nah. 1:12).

There is a limit to affliction, God sends it, and removes it. Do you sigh and say, "When will the end be?" Our Father takes away the rod when His design in using it is fully served.

If the affliction is sent for testing us, it will end when the Lord has made us bear witness to His praise.

We closed by joining hands and singing quietly a song of praise, "Hallelujah." The group disbanded with some reluctance.

That evening, Lee, Kim, Candy, and I listened to a replay of the cassette that had been made that morning at the coffee. Candy was particularly interested. I did not have the courage to observe Lee's facial reactions. Not accustomed to talking to groups about God, I was self-conscious that I was coming across like a preacher lady. Both Lee and I believe that how we *live* the Christian life is far more effective than what we say.

February 17

It was time to drive to the clinic to have my stitches removed and more fluid drained.

Sitting in a chair in the examining room, I had on the now-familiar paper gown that gaps no matter how you wear it. I had chosen the gap-in-the-back style. The door opened slowly and Dr. Allen inquired, "May I use the word . . . uh . . . *ravishing*?" He was not only highly skilled in his field and unusually compassionate and sensitive toward his patients' feelings, but he had a way with words. . . . Every surgical patient should be so lucky.

Dr. Allen showed me a detailed typewritten copy of the surgical procedures that had been performed on me. At the bottom, he called particular attention to a sentence reading, "13 lymph nodes removed; all 13 lymph nodes benign." It looked positively beautiful on paper.

His nurse had me lie on my side. It was obvious that she had been elected chief stitch-puller of the afternoon. During the process, there was little discomfort; the area was still numb. Approximately four stung briefly. However, by the time she came to #31, she shook hands with Mr. Stubborn Stitch. After jabbing unsuccessfully four or five times, she commented in exasperation, "I can't get this one. He put it in; he can take it out."

While this was taking place I was deliberately carrying on a steady stream of dialogue. I had decided ahead of time that if I concentrated on becoming acquainted with the stitch-*puller*, I wouldn't be thinking about the stitches. It worked.

Then Dr. Allen inserted a needle into the incision and fluid rushed out. He asked me to sit up. Upon pushing around the area he noticed that a considerable amount of fluid remained under the skin. He and the nurse compared it to a water bed. Sure enough, you could see the fluid move from one location to another by merely applying pressure. Dr. Allen decided to use a larger needle. This time it gushed forth. The nurse measured 300 ccs. When I stepped on the scale the next morning I weighed two pounds less than I had the day before.

Now I was more comfortable sleeping. I no longer had that taut, stretched feeling. My upper right arm remained tender between the elbow and the shoulder socket, particularly on the inside of the arm. Dr. Allen assured me that this would improve. It was my only source of discomfort. I noticed that if I had an extremely active day, my arm hurt me more that night. It was as though the amount of pain acted as a barometer of the amount of activity that had taken place that day. I decided to slow down.

17

No Bionic Woman

Friday, February 18

My sister, Betty, her husband Newt, their son, Doug, and Rose, a close family friend, arrived from Pennsylvania for the weekend. Betty, born on my fourth birthday, is the sister who lost her leg in an automobile accident. She had been a model of outstanding courage and determination to me.

Newt shared her skill on the squash court. We drove into the Lake Shore Racquet Club in time to watch him defeat his first opponent in the National championships. Before his next scheduled match we had lunch and viewed the sights of the Windy City. We were exhausted when we reached home nearly twelve hours later—particularly me.

Our weekend included sister talk for Betty and me, building blocks for Doug and Scott, and happy humor for Newt and his nieces. I enjoyed fussing a bit, setting a festive table and preparing a special meal on Sunday.

Monday, February 21

Our houseguests pulled out of our driveway in the morning at 10:15. By 10:30 my company nerves were screaming. Kim and Candy were the unfortunate recipients. Having pleaded exhaustion from our exciting weekend, they had received permission to stay home from school to catch up on sleep. Between 10:15 and 10:30 I received three phone calls. At 10:30, while transferring wet laundry from washer to dryer, I noticed the ceiling in the laundry room vibrating. Raucous rock sounds screamed from Candy's eight-track stereo in the room overhead. And *she* needed sleep? I needed sleep. All of me. I craved Peace and Quiet. I exploded. I was not the bionic woman!!!!

We had it out. I made it inordinately clear that I was now doing all of the housework, washing, playing hostess, etc. since Gram had left. It was two and one-half weeks since major surgery and I desperately needed the help of my two teenage daughters. My voice changed from overly polite to hysterical.

Their response was not sympathetic, not positive, not what I wanted to hear. They fled to their father, who played peacemaker. I was ordered to bed where I wept and slept for three hours, a healing experience but also a learning experience. I awoke refreshed, wrote in my journal for hours and visited with Luci.

My sister Ruth called from New Jersey, and we agreed that it might be wiser for me to refrain from more houseguests until I had my full strength. She suggested methods to maintain a quiet center and emphasized the importance of taking things easy—perhaps lowering my expectations.

During this period I was certain a basketball was growing under my right arm. I learned later that the severed nerves were directly related to the nervous system and the tautness and aching sensation under my arm were signals shouting "Slow down." I did. I refused to play model hostess and perfect homemaker.

I learned a valuable lesson, though not soon enough. I had felt good after surgery and was accustomed to being active. However, I was not the same. My nervous system and my body as well were tired, having been through a major ordeal.

After coming home from the hospital I should have remained in my robe and slippers—not jumped into jeans. Because of being so careful with my hair and my makeup, from all outward appearances I didn't look any different. In fact, perhaps I looked better since I had lost weight. To my children I was Wonder Woman. Clues were questions like "Where are my gym clothes? Did you get my white sweater washed? How come we're not having mashed potatoes with the pork chops?" Meantime the phone rang repeatedly, the doorbell continued to chime, toothpaste stuck to the sinks, and thank-you notes needed to be written.

Later in the day I spoke to a Bible study group which was responsive and friendly. I was warmed to see Carolyn there.

Stopping afterwards to purchase a birthday cake for Candy who turned fourteen today, I bumped into Carolyn. We laughed at how God had allowed us to meet. The two of us had been trying to get together for months. We decided to have lunch. I *learned* from simply being with Carolyn.

She too had been through a severe crisis, having attempted suicide when her husband had left her for another woman. While she was in the hospital, her life in the balance, an inner voice had insisted that I go see her and tell her that she must try to live for herself and her two children. Carolyn recovered her desire to continue with life, she reluctantly granted Paul a divorce, and she clung to God for her stability. He did not fail her. After a seemingly endless period of time, Paul returned to Carolyn and their son and daughter and they were remarried at the loveliest, most meaningful ceremony I have witnessed. Both children participated in the service. Carolyn was radiant. I wept unashamedly.

Now, over the table at a restaurant, Carolyn was ministering to me. She shared ways that she was truly loving to her husband. How God was helping her to be more appreciative, more demonstrative, and more sexually aggressive.

"You have so much love for all of these girls with whom

you are sharing your story. Do you have as much for Lee?"
Carolyn gently inquired. "Let's get our homes in order and
truly love the people in our own families. Then we can love
all of those others," she suggested.

I got into our station wagon and soon my favorite radio station was playing "Something Beautiful." God's Spirit was
quieting me. While driving I began to examine my priorities. I forced myself to consider Carolyn's words. I wanted
to be more of a loving wife to Lee, but did I demonstrate as
much love to him as I did to others outside of our home?
Probably not. It was true that I was beginning to respond
to the new Lee more all of the time; however, I was still
nursing hurts that hadn't quite healed in our relationship.
It *was* much easier to sparkle, to quip, to reach out to
people I was with for briefer periods of time. The more I
thought about it the more I became convinced that I did
share my brightest, best self with my friends. I arrived home
to collapse on the couch.

I was to learn more from Carolyn. Some time later I received the following letter.

Dear, dear Janie:

How special today was. Having you visit the store. God is
sure good to me.

Remember I told you I read something from a special book
after having lunch with you that I thought I'd like to share?
Well, here it is. I came home tonight to quiet myself before
Paul, beautiful Paul, arrived home, and decided to quickly put
it on paper. This is from the book *Joy Is* by Gilbert Beers.

APPOINTMENTS

Lord, my appointment book is bulging. There is a luncheon
on Tuesday, crowded in between a half dozen or so business appointments during the day. After dinner I'm scheduled to be at
P.T.A.

Today I had a *minute* to think. That's unusual. A real luxury!
You know that, Lord.

I thought about my appointment book. I looked at the names

in it. Then I felt ashamed. I couldn't find some very important names. The real V.I.P.'s in my life.

Where was my husband's name? I didn't have his down for 3:30 Wednesday afternoon, or luncheon on Monday or an evening of fun and relaxation. No, his name should be up there near the top of the list.

There are some other V.I.P.'s I've missed. My children. Where are they scheduled? They need my time just as these others do. MORE! MUCH MORE! I can see that I need to rework my book and get things in better order.

Oh, how could I forget, Lord? I don't have you in here either. Look at all those other names and dates and places! Not once do I have you down for a Specific Time and Place.

"Meet God at the family room chair at 7:30 a.m. Purpose of meeting: Straighten out priorities. Rearrange appointments, and make sure V.I.P.'s are put in top place."

Lord, help me rearrange my appointments the way they should be.

Joy is putting things in the right perspective.

Love you,
Carolyn

Wednesday, February 23

The setting was the living room of one of the large lovely older homes in Glen Ellyn—the kind with side porches and spacious, airy rooms. Joan, my fun friend with whom I had lunch the day the prognosis *malignant* was announced, was the hostess. Her high-ceilinged living room was wall-to-wall with tennis friends balancing cups of coffee in exchange for their racquets.

As I related my miracle story I observed facial expressions. Some of these included bewilderment, awe, doubt, respect, unbelief, belief, but mostly wonder. Several times their eyes were creased with tears. So were mine. These were the women with whom I had played countless matches in the summer sun. Side by side we would grow tan as our children swam in the turquoise water of the club pool. When I wasn't engrossed in a book, I was exchanging ideas with these, my summer friends. Several of them I was seeing for the first time out of the club costume of tennis dress or swim suit. I loved them, each and every one, and they knew it. These were the girls that had showered me with calls, cards, casseroles, jewelry, concern and a veritable garden of plants and fresh flowers.

I had attempted to live out my Christian faith with them, but before then I had not verbalized it. I believe that Christians need to earn the right to be heard. Now after a sequence of summers building bridges of friendship, the moment had arrived to share my story.

Afterwards, nearly all of them stood quietly in line to embrace me. When Adele hugged me, she whispered, "I am so proud to be one of your friends."

I was drained. But very, very happy. That day I glimpsed one of the reasons God allowed me to experience the trauma of breast cancer. It was so that I could know the joy of sharing Him.

I drove from Joan's to the medical clinic and waited in turn for my weekly checkup with Dr. Allen. Finally, his head peeked around the door. "Billy Jean?"

"No, Chris." I returned his quip.

Fluid was still having to be drained. I peeked as Dr. Allen cautioned me about the large needle that had been inserted into my chest wall. "Don't move or it will be flat against your rib cage."

I moved. I felt it against my rib cage.

When he had finished, Dr. Allen commented, "It's healing nicely. Next week I probably won't have to do this. In fact, I'm going to let you play tennis."

"I want to play with you." I said.

"I'd love to play with you."

Still later, now fully dressed (Dr. Allen had never seen me with my clothes *on*), I tapped him on the shoulder in the corridor and said with a perfectly composed face, "I've just reserved Court 3 at the racquet club at eight o'clock next Wednesday night. We'll begin with doubles. O.K.?" I was joking. I knew he wanted me to wait another week before returning to my favorite sport.

I fairly floated out of there. Unfortunately, because of Dr. Allen's demanding surgical schedule, our tennis date never took place.

Sunday, February 27

After church some of Steve's college friends joined us for pot roast, carrots, potatoes and gravy. Life was returning to normal again. After dinner I couldn't refuse an invitation to play Ping Pong. Lee had built a cozy game room adjoining the horses' stalls. Because it lacked a furnace, he installed a wood-burning stove which the players kept supplied with wood. However, on this frozen February day we didn't burn much wood. We generated our own body heat by the pace of the game. Steve, Kevin, Kim and I were the participants, with Scott and our dog Queen the spectators. The scores were consistently close, the atmosphere competitive. After four games of doubles, I couldn't resist the opportunity to beat Kevin, a husky member of the college football team, in several games of singles.

Monday, February 28

Lee and I enjoyed a special time together. Our relationship was comfortable these days. I was growing more free to be me and he to be himself. On our way home from the automobile show, we stopped at Poppin' Fresh Pies. In this same place, just a month earlier, we had discussed with Marion and Bob how I would feel if I were to learn that the biopsy result was cancer. Again, I was reminded of all that had transpired in so short a time. Lee and I talked about the fact that there were actually periods now when we *forgot* that cancer had been confirmed and eliminated within twenty-four hours. The following journal entry describes how I felt:

Nearly a full day will pass with my being unaware that I am missing a breast. I don't *feel* any different. . . . Yes, I do. Way inside, where my soul and spirit live, I feel freer, liberated, more loved by God. I also feel more loved by Lee, by my children, and by my friends. The sky is bluer, each branch is more distinctly outlined against the sky. Friends' faces— voices—seem warmer, friendlier. I am more aware of others' pain, of others' feelings, and of others' non-verbal signals of communication. I also have an increased ability to unload my problems, struggles and anxieties to God. I want to be in touch with Him on a regular basis. I am more interested in discovering what He wants. Whom shall I write to today, call today, be home for today?

On Friday, March 4, none of our children had school. All four pitched in to clean the house for the twenty ladies who were coming at one o'clock. Steve vacuumed, Lee scrubbed the foyer, and Kim and Candy did their Saturday chores a day early. We were a team, making our home sparkle. A day earlier, through the front window I had noticed two nursery-men digging around our shrubs and mulching the trees. The yard was receiving a spring cleanup. I looked again and recognized them—Lee and Steve.

The talk went well. Again, I could read a variety of expressions as I spoke. An approving nod, a warm responsiveness, a skeptical stare. . . .

A few days later I received this note from one of those present:

Dear Janie:
What a brave thing you did—you were so moved with your experiences you wanted to share them.

What stands out in my mind is the value of good, strong friendships in your hour of need to help you accept. How lucky you are for friends like Joan, Marion and Katie.

As you know, some people did not accept what you said, but in *their* hour of need they might remember what you said—and that's all you can hope for.

Mary Ann

The next day Katie, my riding friend, and I rode horseback beneath a blue, blue sky. The sun shone warm against our faces. It felt good to be in the saddle. I held the reins with my left hand. Blaze and Brandy were spirited and as happy as we to be riding the trail again.

Later I shared a concern with Lee. Perhaps I was coming on too strong in my talks. Too religious.

That afternoon a letter arrived that eased my anxiety. To Lee and to me it was another example of God's incredible timing.

Dear Janie,

I've just returned home and you're very much on my mind!

Of course, you *look* simply marvelous! But I saw inside you an awe-inspiring loveliness and a "light" which truly reflects God's love that you shared with us today! I am humbled and oh so grateful for being included. . . .

I can identify with some of the "mechanics" of your hospitalization—like your roommate, and those meaningful prayers asking God to help us—just to cope and adjust! You did strike many a "nerve" with me—and I can't begin to tell you how very much stronger I feel because of your sharing! . . .

Your experience—which is still going on—is incredibly profound to me! I commend you for being able to give of yourself so freely—and yet *very* low-key religiously—so that so many can participate!! . . .

Yes, the same God who is with you is with me—we might wear the mantle a little differently which I believe is part of God's plan—but we're all different anyway—and I just want you to know I think you're a treasure here on earth! . . .

I guess I could sum up everything I feel in asking you to refer to Romans 1:11–12. Am *not* one to quote Scripture openly—but this is a *very* special one for me. I thank *you*, Janie Clausen, for being refreshed by you!

God bless you, Lee, and your lovely family!

Affectionately,
Joanie Z.

P.S. You've made me aware of the *necessary* "clinical" check. I shall do this! Thanks, chum!

18

Breasts and Sex after Surgery

Three weeks after my mastectomy our entire family went roller skating with a group from church. This was an activity we had enjoyed for years. As I whirled around I felt myself being stared at by one of the men, a retiring ministerial student. Before long, he skated up to me and inquired how I was feeling. His eyes were riveted to my chest. Back and forth they moved, from one breast to another. I imagined him asking, "Would the real breast please stand up?" I made a mental note to look for a large button I could pin to my left chest which read, "I am the REAL ONE." I did not help him in his dilemma. I didn't know how. It was amusing.

I continued to find it amusing as other men skated up and greeted me, their eyes moving downward to my snug sweater (I had borrowed it from Candy). I caught up to Lee and told him about this new phenomenon. Before long Steve skated by and did a mock imitation of the same performance. Lee overexaggerated his interpretation, moving his eyes back and forth on my sweater, a questioning look on his face, all the while carrying on a steady stream of conversation unrelated to the subject.

Lee and I executed some synchronized skating to a Barry Manilow song. The lights were low, the mood was romantic, the evening an unexpected delight. Our children told us later that we had shown off on the Couples Only selections. We chose to ignore this comment.

Discovering that I was able to skate again was gratifying. It gave me confidence that other sports would soon again be possible for me. However, I did notice swelling and accumulation of fluid that evening when I undressed for bed.

After the lights were out I reflected on the evening. Why had the male skaters been staring at my breasts? It made me angry. They could have asked me how I was feeling—but no, it appeared that my altered appearance mattered more.

The symbol of the breast in American culture has become all-pervasive. It has been used to sell cars, magazines, and detergent. Even television in recent years has begun offering programs that are nothing more than exploitive chest shots. Imagine a society that lights its cigarets from matchbooks that show a closeup shot of a woman's breasts with the slogan "Quebec and Canada—so good together, why separate them?"

No wonder American men and woman are preoccupied with breasts. For the sake of profit, TV, the movie industry, slick advertising all promote the obsession. Consider the attention placed on the mammary glands of Jane Russell, Marilyn Monroe, Farah Fawcett Majors, Bo Derek and others too numerous to name. How can a woman *not* feel that the size of her breasts is important? With girlie magazines flooding the newsstands it is only natural to feel inadequate if you do not measure at least a 34B. Even one of the popular sports magazines features a section on skintight, see-through swim suits in a special annual edition. Lee's American Nurseryman magazine advertises power mowers pushed by beautiful girls with bulging breasts.

A little more than five years ago, a New York couple, Daphne Ayalah and Isaac Weinstock, asked 300 women to take off their clothes and—without the benefit of makeup or soft lighting or glamorous settings—offer their breasts to Ayalah's camera. And 300 women did. The result, a book, *Breasts: Women Speak About Their Breasts and Their Lives*—a sometimes funny, often sad account of the state of the breast in a breast-crazed culture. I read about this in a *Chicago Tribune* article by Ann Marie Lipinski. She reported a comment by Ayalah that men aren't the only ones with a fetish for "perfect" breasts. "Women are also very concerned," she said, "with what they feel is just the right size and form; if given the chance they'll almost always find something to criticize. They'll say they're too small or too large, too round or too pendulous, too high or too low, or not perfectly even. They never think of their breasts as just *there*, like toes or kneecaps, or whatever."

This obsession is fueled every time a woman wheels her shopping cart through a checkout line, says Weinstock, who is thirty-two. "She looks over her shoulder only to see a copy of *Cosmopolitan*, complete with a full-color photo of a woman whose breasts can hardly be contained on the cover. Everywhere she goes she's bombarded with these images to the point where it's hard to feel anything *but* inadequate."

Ayalah admitted she was as much a product of this breast-obsessed culture as anyone. Working on the book, however, made her feel much better about her breasts, and she hopes her readers will feel better too. Her discovery that a lot of women have breasts that are subtly lopsided, made it easy for her to admit that hers were too. "Having seen so many women's breasts, I now fully accept the size that I am and the shape that I am," she said. "I also feel much less frightened by the possibility of breast cancer. Having been subjected to so many women who have had mastectomies, I feel prepared, I feel on top of it. I feel as though I have already dealt with much of the psychic trauma."

The breasts that sell in the slick advertising world were usually made-up, propped-up, airbrushed images that were long on fantasy but short on truth. Real breasts just didn't look that way, the authors reasoned.

It is easy for women to become locked into the opinion that the size and shape of our breasts is significant. On the other hand, perhaps we should become more concerned with what *we are,* what our value and priorities are, rather than how we look. To quote Lee, "The depths of a man's love for his wife doesn't depend on the size of her breasts."

A man falls in love with more than a woman's body. He falls in love with the real you, the whole you, with your sense of humor, and with the life you and he share together. Your ability to love, to give of yourself, and to sparkle are all a part of a man's love for his woman.

As far as the sexual relationship is concerned, I asked myself, what makes the difference as to whether or not a couple's sex life is affected following a mastectomy?

According to one psychologist, the worst problem between husbands and wives is misunderstanding. Sometimes the husband would like to be considerate and not press the wife about sex. The wife might interpret this as a loss of desire on his part. The biggest problem is not how the husband feels but *how the woman feels about herself.* Age has nothing to do with it. Vanity may—or perhaps insecurity. And security has nothing to do with the pieces of you; it has to do with the total you.

I have come to the conclusion that how happy I feel about myself is in direct relation to how much happiness I experience on a daily level. If I am unhappy with who I am, I am more likely to be unhappy with the significant others in my life. On the other hand, if I like who I am, and, if I can accept my limitations realistically, I can do the same for others.

Jesus says in Matthew 22:39, Mark 12:31, and Luke 10:27 that we should love our neighbors as ourselves. In other words, self-love is thus the prerequisite and criterion for our conduct towards our neighbor. The Bible confirms what modern psychology has discovered: without self-love, there can be no love for others.

Before I had my surgery, I liked myself and felt comfortable inside my skin. After my mastectomy the day arrived when I finally took a long look at the neat pink scar where my breast had been. I still felt comfortable with the me that

was *inside* my skin. I reasoned that "it was still the same
me." And, if I was missing one less outside ornament, how
could this alter the basic, honest-to-goodness me? My husband, family, and friends never loved me for my two breasts.
Consequently, their love would not be changed—certainly
not be made less. Loving someone means loving the whole
person, inside and out. Beauty is only skin deep. Lee's love
was not based on my outside physical body. He did not love
me any less—perhaps more. His constant visits to the hospital, his genuine concern and support, and his tenderness
convinced me of this. Therefore, I reasoned, why should *I*
feel less comfortable about me?

I chose to accept my new, slightly altered physical body
and determined not to allow it to interfere with our sex life.
It didn't. The very night I arrived home from the hospital I
lifted the loose bandage on my chest and asked Lee to take a
look at it. I watched his eyes carefully. They didn't flinch. A
bit of confidence that things would be O.K. moved into my
mind. While getting ready for bed or into my swimsuit I
forced myself to undress and to walk unselfconsciously without clothing from our walk-in closet to the bathroom and
bedroom. I wanted Lee to become accustomed to the new
lopsided me. He did. He affirmed me. He assured me that
the sight of one side of my chest flat did not affect his physical desire for me. This was confirmed by the fact that our
lovemaking was not affected.

I believe that having satisfying sex is essential for marital
happiness. More than before, I wanted to make my man
happy. More than ever I needed the reassurance that he
found me an attractive bed companion. No way was I going
to allow the loss of one breast to interfere with our sex life.
Too much was at stake. By this time, having been married
twenty-four years, I knew that a husband values a warm, responsive sexual companion more than a wife with a Barbie
doll figure. I was right.

As the days passed, I felt that I had not so much lost as

gained something—a deeper appreciation for the gift of life, for the inestimable value of friends, and for the genuine caring of my family. I also gained a deeper faith in the sovereignty of God and experienced the enormous rewards of a simple deep faith. Those five days in the hospital when I trusted His strength, God rewarded me richly. He gave me an awareness of His presence, the conviction that He was working out His purposes in both my life and the lives of others, and an indescribable peace. Combined with these was a sense of expectancy that He would see me through *anything* that developed.

Recently I heard Dr. Stuart Briscoe say on the radio, "Expose every situation to the adequacy of Christ." When I put this suggestion into practice, I have discovered less pressure and anxiety in living.

It helps to have a sense of humor about our breasts—and ourselves. My friend Katie made this graphic for me with a couple of phone calls before and after my surgery. A quip a day helps keep depression away. . . .

The first call went something like this: "Are you ready for this, Janie? Stan always says that a boob in the hand is worth two in the bush. Just think about that, and be sure to tell Lee."

And then this, a day or two later: "Are you ready? For forty-four years you have had a cleavage on the tennis court, and frankly, I'm sick of it. I have never had one and will never have one. It's time that you lose half of that cleavage. . . ."

I howled. Her remarks helped me to keep things in their perspective. How important was it *really* whether I had one or two boobs? The fact that I was free of cancer and had my *life* was of far more worth.

19

Tennis, Anyone?

I learned the hard way that major surgery saps a patient's strength and that one will feel tired for several weeks—even months—afterwards. Exactly five weeks after my mastectomy I returned to my job at the college. It was a neat treat to be bear hugged by one of the men teachers—a distinguished, conservative professor of literature. Meals furnished by friends on two nights were welcome and more helpful than I knew. By Friday afternoon, the fourth eight-hour workday, I was inexpressibly weary and close to tears when the department chairman cautioned me regarding the danger of overdoing my activities. I drove home and succumbed to exhaustion. Tears streaked my cheeks as I collapsed into bed where Lee served me supper. I slept for twelve uninterrupted hours.

On March 17, during my checkup, Dr. Allen announced, "You look great. You don't need to come back. *You may begin playing tennis again.*" I returned to my office and reserved a court for 8:00 P.M. that evening.

I was apprehensive when Lee sent the first couple of balls over the net. However, soon I was stroking the ball with increasing confidence. Wow! Did it feel good to be moving on the court again. At first, my shots resembled a beginner's, but I was soon stepping into the ball and placing it with a degree of accuracy.

At nine o'clock my sense of gratitude was profound. Exactly six weeks earlier I had had major surgery, a breast and lymph nodes removed on my right side, and here I was, cured of that dreaded disease, cancer, hitting the tennis ball again, with the encouragement of my husband.

When we returned to the darkened privacy of our car, I lifted my heart to God with thankfulness.

The following day I experienced no muscular soreness. Though my strength was gradually returning, my work schedule continued to be taxing. Temporarily I had to give up the speaking sessions, and by Easter, I had decided to leave my job at the end of the term—two weeks later, April 18.

A week before Easter, Lee had had a brief heart flare-up. Easter Sunday itself had special meaning as we reflected on all the ways in which God had blessed us. Two days earlier, on Good Friday, one of our friends, Lee's age, dropped dead of a heart attack on a Florida beach. It could have been Lee. . . .

On Easter the temperature soared into the eighties and the sky shouted with sunshine. An egg hunt began the day. After church and Sunday dinner we dispersed to do our own thing: Scott and I to the lawn chairs with current books, Kim and Candy to saddle their horses, and Steve and Lee to watch sports on TV.

Later, Steve and I paired up against Kim and Candy for two sets of tennis, the girls hitting the ball with smooth, polished strokes. At three o'clock Lee and Steve's friend, Dave, appeared for the Big Match. The two recently confined hospital victims had issued a challenge to the two college boys; Steve and Dave were two of our favorite opponents. Rackets swung, the ball flew back and forth over the net and, as usual, the game scores were close. Finally, the elder doubles pair captured two sets.

Later, as the sun dropped from sight, we reluctantly went indoors. Warmed by the sun and good feelings, Lee and I crowded close in our oversized bed to watch "Jesus of Nazareth" on TV. We felt fortunate that we were acquainted with this unique Man who was responsible for the first Easter.

On my last day at the college, Linda, a literature major, stopped by and we got to talking about changes, my hospital adventure, and the importance of being willing to be used for our Lord. Afterwards, I was struck silent when she accompanied herself on the guitar she was carrying and sang of how endings can become beginnings. I couldn't help thinking of the imminent termination of my job in the English Department. Linda's dark eyes met mine as she sang, and I was conscious of how we were united in that moment in our awareness of God's potential in our lives. I identified with her search and the longing expressed in the words she had written. A search for a tangible God. For direction. For a singleness of purpose. For serenity.

Serenity was in short supply on a June Sunday several weeks later. Rick, our church's youth director, loved to play tennis. His wife, Kori, and I loved to ride horseback. We had been trying to get our families together for swimming, tennis, and a picnic. Finally we found a day. Kori and their three children were in the pool when it happened. Lee and I were changing sides of the tennis court when Steve sent a sizzling warmup serve over the net that caught me dead center in my left eye. I never saw the ball. I didn't even get my eyelid closed. The impact knocked me off my feet. The pain was severe. My eye smarted, closed halfway, and teared continuously. But we had waited so long for this get-together with the Lane family that I wasn't about to have it interrupted. I returned to the court and played four more sets.

Following a pleasant picnic supper and more swimming and tennis, we decided to call it a day. By the time we reached home, my eye was very uncomfortable. Lee drove me to an eye clinic where an ophthalmologist told me that I

was a very lucky lady. It seems that my eye had hemor-
rhaged internally and then had miraculously formed a clot in
spite of the fact that I continued to play. The doctor firmly
ordered me to bed where I must have both eyes bandaged. I
must remain *perfectly still* for five days with only bathroom
privileges. I was not to uncover either eye or get out of bed
for five days!! I had received a hard wallop and if the clot dis-
solved (tore lose) I could lose the sight in my left eye. He
recommended that Lee place me in the hospital where I
would be closely supervised. Above all else, I *must* remain
still.

The news hit hard. In the quietness of that darkened office
I closed my eyes and cried. It didn't make matters any better
that both Lee and the doctor sat without words and witnessed the wet tears sliding down my cheeks. Why was I
taking it so hard? I didn't know. Dr. Douglas inquired
whether I had cried during my recent confinement for
cancer. When I answered "no," he concluded that this was a
delayed reaction. I resented his arrogant analyzing and chose
not to explain to him my wondrous adventure in the hospital
and afterwards.

Armed with a prescription for valium, I returned to our
bed with an attitude of resignation and some anger. I was
disappointed in myself that I had not accepted the doctor's
prognosis with serenity. Where was this inner quiet I had
talked and written about? Had He, the Source of serenity,
deserted me?

I had five days to think, listen to music, talk with friends
on the phone, and rediscover His quiet caring.

Thursday, four days after the accident, I received permission to remove both bandages for a special occasion, Candy's
graduation from eighth grade. Her lithe, athletic figure was
slightly out of focus as she walked down the center aisle of
the crowded gym carrying a single long-stemmed rose. She
resembled more angel than athlete in her sister's long ivory
lace trimmed dress, her tawny wedge haircut a shining cap
on her head.

When it was Candy's turn to step forward to the podium to read a poem emphasizing the importance of a smile, my vision was foggy. The latter was not due to having caught a tennis ball in my eye, but the blur of tears.

Throughout my days of confinement Lee exercised great patience and good humor with me. He carefully changed the dressings over my eyes and administered the required number of drops. On more than one occasion the goop from the medicine stuck to the gauze, making it difficult to remove the bandage. Lee tenderly softened the area with warm water to avoid any discomfort for me. Through encounters like this I was reminded that my husband possessed a quality that most women, including me, valued enormously: tenderness. The tension in our relationship was becoming less visible, and I found myself responding to his gentleness and sensitivity.

An interesting phenomenon was taking place. God was doing a thorough job of healing. First, he healed Lee in August in Jamaica, 1974. The result, a changed man who made an about-face in his attitude toward what was important in life. He changed from being self-pitying, defensive, and undisciplined to become a self-respecting, faithful family man.

God healed me of fear and anxiety regarding the consequences of cancer and then placed me on the path to a radical recovery following surgery. During this critical time, He began healing me of painful memories, bitterness, and a vindictive spirit toward those who had hurt me. He replaced my negative attitude with one that included love and forgiveness. He then supplied me with a strong sense of self-identity, a singleness of purpose, and the ability to respond to my husband again. Suspicion was replaced with trust, disfavor with respect, and depression with a delicious sense of expectancy.

Two weeks after my eye injury I picked up a severe case of sinusitis. For a period of three weeks I was drugged with fatigue and medication, my body attempting to fight the infection. I asked God why I had to be set aside a third time.

He seemed to say, "Be still, my child. Be still."

The tennis racket rested more—and so did I. Not feeling up to housework or tennis, I turned instead to writing and to enriching relationships. While Lee fished in Canada with the three older children, I spent time touching in with friends on a one-to-one basis. Always, always blowing my nose and clearing my throat. Afternoons by the pool became talk sessions. Unknown bathing-suit-clad figures became persons with names, needs, distinctive personalities—new friends. Each one needed to be listened to—to be loved. The sight of Scott's sturdy, sun-bronzed body in his striped swim-trunks became a familiar sight as I wrote and reflected by the pool.

What *was* really important?

What about sex? It seemed that every magazine I picked up featured either articles or advertisements of books emphasizing the importance of the sexual experience. Never had history placed such an emphasis on the orgasm. Sex had become the *summum bonum* of life. I reminded myself that love, not sex, is the basic need for each of us. I thought more about this and came to the conclusion that the more I focused on the goodness and the love of God to me, the more I was enabled to love others. I noticed that having an attitude of faith, which went beyond me, fastened my attention on larger purposes. I needed to get my approval, my sense of being loved and worthwhile, from Him, not from the response of those around me.

My thoughts continued in this vein. Throughout my crisis with cancer, God had demonstrated immeasurable kindness to me as well as provided me with a quiet center from which to navigate. It appeared that the snags and spaces in our marriage were slowly but surely on the mend. My chances for a complete recovery from cancer were excellent. Yes, I had much for which to be grateful. I had a large supply of love and light and joy inside to spread around. I now had a sense of personal worth for which I had been seeking so long. I wanted to be present in every moment of life—feeling it, enjoying it, learning, exploring, appreciating the world God made and the people in it. I was alive to my senses. "Life is a daring adventure . . . or it is nothing" (Helen Keller).

After sifting these thoughts into my computer, I again asked myself, *What is really important?* Having a no-cellulite figure with shapely breasts? Winning tournament tennis matches? Keeping a clean, shining house? No. Again I arrived at the same conclusion I had reached in the hospital. Building relationships. Reaching out and touching. Taking each day as a fresh new gift to live out His love.

20

The Missing Ingredient

By July the summer routine was well established. There were swimming and tennis lessons for Scott and tennis team practice for Candy. I was playing in two round-robin tournaments, one of them mixed doubles with Steve as my partner. There was little to remind me of my mastectomy except for an occasional puffy soreness in the area of my right armpit. I noticed this more after tennis and planned to switch to a lightweight racket.

It was delicious to experience again that familiar thwock of the ball as it hit the strings. Winning wasn't quite as important as it had been other summers. Playing well was. Losing graciously was. Maintaining a warm, encouraging relationship with the others on the court was.

Kim and I were looking over the summer sales. I selected two swimsuits. Kim, a smart shopper, was watching me pirouette in front of the mirror. I was trying to choose between a colorful green dressmaker style and a blue two-piece. (The latter would be my first two-piece suit ever.) One symbolized middle age, modesty, mastectomy; the other, a daring, refreshing, new, why-not-try-me look. The saleswoman thought the vivid green one looked great with my tan, but I decided on the latter. The two-piece turned out to be a success in spite of the fact that I nearly lost it twice while riding ocean waves later in the summer. Lee and the children applauded my choice.

The first two weeks of August our annual family reunion was held. Equipped with a new wedge haircut and a figure that was slimmer by ten pounds, I set off for the southern tip of New Jersey with the three younger children.

Our destination was Cape May, a charming seaside town with interesting old clapboard hotels and a flower-bedecked shopping mall to delight the rainy-day shopper.

For years my dad had been gathering his four daughters, his son, and their respective families to vacation together. It got so that each of the cousins, along with their parents, would count the days until the annual Woll family reunion. From as far as southern California, Florida, Illinois, New Jersey and Pennsylvania we assembled to touch in—to laugh, play, and sometimes cry together. Through the months between reunions, letters, notes, snapshots, books and phone calls were exchanged informing members of various circumstances and events. No matter how traumatic a difficulty that might occur in one of the families, the others would quickly lend their assistance and affirmation. It was always there, that silent support. That reaching out across the miles that separated us to care, to be available in time of need and in time of celebration.

I was looking forward to the gathering of the clan this year even more than usual. Perhaps it was because it would be the first time I would be with members of my own family since I had faced cancer and possible death. On the last occasion we were together, I had discovered the disturbing discharge. It had been in Florida, just seven months earlier.

Lee and Steve were going to join us at the beginning of the second week of our vacation. For the third consecutive summer I drove, and we made our customary stop overnight in Youngstown, Ohio. However, this time Kim, just turned sixteen, was able to share the driving. While she took her turn at the wheel, I raced through the pages of the recently

published *First, You Cry* by Betty Rollin. In this intimate,
incredibly frank story Betty tells how the loss of a breast affects her emotions, her sex life, her job, her feelings, and
her femininity. It was engrossing—and a unique opportunity
to find out how another woman had reacted to this major
event. *First, You Cry* held me, gripped and moved me.

Instead of waiting in line for hamburgers at turnpike gas
stops, we selected a slice of shade where we consumed sub-
marine sandwiches, fruit, and Pepsi. A thoughtfully packed
freezer chest was a common passenger on family trips.
Sometimes we pulled over at waysides to stretch our stiff
muscles by playing Simon Says and running relays. I kept a
pillow and quilt close by for snatches of shuteye and sun
soaking. To add interest to the endless miles we played word
games and Twenty Questions. I challenged the children to
invent titles to the lush scenery on display through the car
windows. Some of their suggestions, particularly in the roll-
ing hills of western Pennsylvania, particularly appealed to
me—"God's Window," "Shades of Green," and "Patterns of
Praise."

When I saw my sister Ruth I clasped her in my arms. As
"my Bobbsey twin at the seashore" and I hugged each other,
our authentic and not authentic breasts complemented each
other, her left breast and my right having been removed. It
was healthy and consoling to be able to laugh about our missing parts.

More magic memories were made at Cape May that summer of '77—strolls beside the ocean, hearing my niece sing a
special song (dedicated to me) at a supper club where she
waitressed, playing hours of tennis daily, sunning on beach
chairs by the sea, and riding the waves in with my brother
and sisters like carefree children. Since I hadn't yet purchased a prosthesis, I stuffed a tennis sock into the right cup
of my new two-piece swim suit. The Atlantic Ocean now has
several unmatched tennis socks in its collection of underwa-
ter treasures.

Before the second week began, Steve and Lee arrived to complete our gang and to be included in the making of family memories that would linger long in our minds. My immediate family was complete now; and I was more complete. At times there were as many as sixteen of our clan stroking the favorite yellow tennis ball on the clay courts in town. Everyone was familiar with the game, including trim and tan Granddad Woll, his five married children and their spouses, and all twenty of the grandchildren. It was with joy that I was able to enter in fully with these family tennis matches, and to know that my game had not suffered. In fact, it was stronger. When the four sisters paired up to play against each other, I was able to hold my own.

I was thankful. We all were.

One nagging ache kept cropping up, however. Throughout the summer I was aware of an invisible wall which prevented me from loving Lee without reservations. Much as I tried to will and pray it away, it remained. Noticing that we had several major arguments at Cape May, my brother, Jim, and his wife, Carol, recommended that Lee and I begin meeting with a therapist on a weekly basis. They had met with one in southern California weekly for a year and a half. As a result, they discovered that they were more equipped to deal with their differences, more able to handle conflict. We decided to act on their advice and asked Jim and Carol to see if their psychotherapist could recommend one for us located in the Chicago area.

One week later, while driving home on the turnpike in western Pennsylvania, I had a significant experience. Lee and the children were asleep in the back of the station wagon. It was a singularly snug feeling, being the only one awake, surrounded by my sleeping family and the luscious scenery. A favorite recording was playing on the tape deck— B. J. Thomas singing "Hallelujah." I lifted my heart to God in praise and my voice to join B. J.'s.

I began reviewing the wondrous things God had done for

me in the hospital. I thanked Him again and then again. I asked Him whether He could remove that nameless wall that made it difficult for me to express my love to Lee as I had in earlier years. I had asked Him countless times in the past to help me regain that very special feeling for my husband. There had been granted no enabling power. Only a void. Why didn't He do it for me? A verse from the Bible commands us to call on God for those things we have not been able to accomplish in our own power. "For I can do everything God asks me to with the help of Christ who gives me the strength and power" (Phil. 4:13).

I searched my conscious mind. It occurred to me that a necessary ingredient was missing. The essential ingredient I held in my hands in the hospital. *Faith.* Down deep within my inner person I never fully believed that God could do this for me—put the magic back into our marriage. I simply had to make it happen. I had tried, and tried, and tried. It had been my companion too long—the undefined barrier. I was beginning to believe that it was to be permanent. And after all, I had so much for which to be thankful; why should I complain? The lines had fallen to me in pleasant places. I had a lovely home; a kind, unselfish husband; four healthy, responsible children; and a multitude of friends. And yet I wasn't able to love my husband the way he deserved. On the other hand, how many of my friends had a storybook marriage? A deeply loving relationship? Very few. Who was I to think that I must have this?

I continued my contemplation as the miles diminished between Philadelphia and Chicago that evening at twilight on the turnpike. I recalled that God had given me a glorious sense of expectancy during those days both before and following surgery. Why couldn't that same God give me that same gift again? It was then that I chose to *believe fully,* for the first time, that He could. But I had to do my part. Believe. In Mark 11:24 Jesus said to his disciples: "If you only have faith in God your command will be obeyed. All that's required is that you really believe and have no doubt! Listen to me! You can pray for anything, and if you believe, you have it; it's yours!"

I, too, was one of His disciples. I chose to believe. I exercised faith. By this time tears were dripping onto my knit shirt. Who cared? I believed God again.

And that incredible sense of expectancy had returned. What's more, the ugly, undefined wall vanished.

The date was August 15, 1977.

I decided not to tell Lee about the unusual encounter I had with God in the car. I wanted to see whether he would be able to notice a difference in our relationship. I have thought a lot about how I was able to tell that a hideous, long-time monster had vanished. Words are inadequate. I simply know that from that time on (it's been five years) I was given the ability to focus on the plus parts of Lee's personality. The negative aspects—which I had seen as glaringly evident—seemed unimportant now. It was as though I didn't have to work at this. Before, I had discovered myself making a conscious effort to be pleasant and what had resulted was an unnatural politeness. Now, I actually liked him. I wanted to spend time with him, to be close to him, to have sex with him.

I am a night person and Lee is a morning person. Now, instead of remaining up to read, I went to bed at the same time Lee did. Before, when we were in bed I would be thinking, "Why doesn't *he* reach out and take me in his arms?" (I discovered later that he was thinking the same thing, only waiting for *me* to make the first move.) Now, I found myself spontaneously moving over to Lee's side of the bed and maneuvering naturally into the circle of his arms. This was entirely out of character for me.

Before, whenever we argued, we each took offense ever so easily, and I would retreat or withdraw in silence, the issue unresolved. Our defenses would spring into place on a moment's notice. We each were determined to prove that the other was wrong. Now, there didn't seem to be nearly as much about which to quibble. Issues that formerly provoked arguments seemed unimportant now.

It was as though scales had been removed from my eyes and I now saw Lee as the loving, unselfish, sensitive person that he was. He was now easy to love, where before it had become a chore. He hadn't changed; my ability to perceive him had changed. And I believe that God granted me that ability.

There was a new honesty and freedom between us. My journal entry continued:

> Last night we held each other for a long time, touching with great tenderness. It was magic. Storybook reality. Our lovemaking was meaningful. My attitude has changed. I now believe all things are possible. I am falling in love with my husband again.

This, to me, is a greater miracle than the miracle of no pain after breast surgery. God performed spiritual surgery and removed a gigantic obstacle that prevented me from loving my husband. Why didn't God perform this surgery sooner? I don't know. His timing is different from mine. Perhaps it's because it took me so long to believe that He could. And then, when I finally believed, He gave me back my love for Lee. He is my miracle God. For the person who believes, all things are possible.

When Dinie and I ended our round-robin tournament season the preceding week by defeating the number one seed and her partner, assuring ourselves of a first-place trophy, it felt marvelous. But the feeling was hollow and pale compared to the climate of closeness I'd experienced that night with Lee. It had been a long, long time since we had known such unity of spirit and body.

21

Another Biopsy!

The next morning brought a different kind of surprise. It had been six months since my last checkup, and I had an appointment with Dr. Bork for a breast examination and a Pap smear. After a thorough exam, to my complete amazement, the doctor notified me that he had discovered a lump in my left breast. He added that it should be removed immediately. I was stunned. Examining my left breast for lumps had become an automatic procedure and this was the second time within a year that I had been unable to discover an existing lump! This one, as the last, was small and hard. Where the last one was located deep beneath the right breast and well into the layers of tissue, this one was immediately below the nipple, and it moved. Dr. Bork suggested that I not bother with a mammogram but went on to say that it should come out regardless of what a mammogram revealed. He had his nurse call my surgeon immediately for an appointment. The earliest one available was 11:15 the following Wednesday morning, *seven days away!*

I was devastated. I simply could not believe what I had just learned. Part of me wanted to scream. I sat on a stool in the corner of the examining room and cried. Dr. Bork, who was not our regular doctor, stood with his arms crossed waiting for me to collect myself. I left the office, stunned.

When I reached my car I noticed my Bible resting on the front seat. I opened it and my eyes fastened on the seventh and eighth verses of Psalm 138 (LB):

Though I am surrounded by troubles, you will bring me safely through them. You will clench your fist against my angry enemies! Your power will save me. The Lord will work out his plans for my life—for your lovingkindness, Lord, continues forever. Don't abandon me—for you made me.

Again I claimed God's presence, His strength, His inner quiet.

For the most part I was able to relax in Him. I had made arrangements earlier to have lunch with a friend and attend a Bible study that afternoon. I shared the news with Kathy as we divided a club sandwich and her smile supported me. At the Bible study, later, I prayed silently that I would be willing to relate of God's infinite care for me during the last months. It seems that He heard. They listened without moving to how the Lord had been unfailingly present in the past days and months, and God poured an awareness of His Spirit into that small living room. A time of prayer followed. As before, a sense of expectancy came to me, to see how God would use this to work out His purposes.

We had plans to attend a formal Wheaton College function that evening at a local country club and were going to be with a number of college classmates we hadn't seen for twenty-five years. I told myself that if I gave in to the tears that were fighting to escape from behind my lids, my eyes would become puffy and red for the evening event. My vanity kept them inside . . . until Lee walked in the house. They spilled over as I told him about the lump Dr. Bork had discovered that morning.

I loved what he did next. He picked up the phone and arranged for Dr. Allen to check the lump the following morning at the hospital. Now that's what you call taking charge of the situation.

I dressed in party clothes, fastened a smile on my face, and determined to make the most of the evening. It was neat to see and talk with friends we had been with in college so many years earlier. We sat at a table with three fellows with whom Lee had played football and who had lived at Lee's parents' home, a mile off campus. Each had been a part of the flavor of our romance. I couldn't help wondering if they had heard that I had had a mastectomy and what they would think if they knew that I might be facing another one. Dale, Willy, Don, and Lee had been an integral part of the "pony" backfield of their football team and their coach, Willis Gale, was being elected into the Wheaton College Hall of Fame. The occasion turned out to be a pleasant distraction from thinking about the lousy lump in my breast.

November 11, 1977—From my journal

It is 10:15 and I am waiting in the emergency room at the hospital for Dr. Allen. He is going to examine the lump that Dr. Bork discovered yesterday. I think I am calm. However, as many times as I have made the trip to this hospital, I did find myself on the wrong road. My thoughts are racing ahead in time and space. It will be great to see Dr. Allen again. How fast can *he* find the lump? Will it feel malignant to him? Even now, knowing its location, I have trouble finding it. I am more nervous than I care to admit. When the girl at the reception desk asked for my driver's license I discovered it was not in my purse. She told me that she recently learned that she had cancer of the cervix. She hadn't had a Pap smear in six years. When I told her that I might have cancer again, she commented, "I like your attitude. Mine's kind of crummy."

The waiting continued. I overheard someone else describe a friend who was recovering from cancer of the throat. Anger consumed me. When were they going to discover a cure for the Big C? Or, better, discover a prevention of cancer.

More waiting. A pleasant-looking man who was also waiting had been kicked in the head by his horse. I learned that
he was brushing his half-broken quarter horse, holding on to
this halter, when the horse reared. The man clubbed him
with the grooming brush. The horse reared again and kicked
his owner on the top of his head, placing two ugly gashes on
his face. (The horse had not been secured to the fence with a
lead rope.)

I glanced at my watch for the twentieth time. Where is
Dr. Allen? I had haircuts scheduled at noon for both Candy
and me.

By eleven o'clock the waiting room was filled with waiting
people. Their expressions were similar. Tired, anxious, troubled. At times life appears to be a series of interruptions.

A familiar figure in white hurried into the crowded room,
his eyes scanning the group. It was Dr. Allen and he was
looking for me! As I moved quickly toward him he took my
arm and said, "How good it is to see you again. However, I
never wanted it to be under these circumstances."

We approached an empty examining room and my escort
inquired of a nearby nurse if we could use it. She smiled a
yes. "Is the lump in the area of the incision?" he asked with
genuine concern in his voice. He appeared immensely relieved when I answered that it was in the left breast.

"I'll wait outside while you undress."

This struck me as amusing. "Why?" I asked. "I'll simply
pull off my sweater and bra. You've seen me undressed
before."

While his fingers probed expertly, the silence in the small
room was deafening. My eyes never left his face and I was
relieved when his features appeared to relax.

"I don't think this lump is one to worry about."

He probed longer. Finally, he announced with authority.
"I'm going to remove it."

"Why?" I asked.

"Because," he paused, "it's there. And you and I both

need to know for sure. I'll remove it Tuesday under major anesthetic."

"I am scheduled to play tennis for Glen Ayre's traveling team on Wednesday. Should I get a substitute?"

"No. I'll keep the incision small," he said, with his marvelous smile, and hurried off to his next surgical appointment.

My heart lifted. Dr. Allen, my expert surgeon, was not worried about this one. Candy and I made it to the beauty parlor on time for our haircuts which were followed by a gigantic grocery shopping and little time to think. The three older children, Candy, Steve, and Kim, needed to be ready to leave for a weekend in Rockford, and Saturday I was involved in a whirl of housecleaning and preparation for friends who were coming to dinner. In spite of the too-much-to-do day, worry about the lump remained in my subconscious. I wondered about its structure. Could it be malignant? Was I going to continue to develop suspicious lumps? When were these faith-testing incidents going to end? I relinquished the despicable lump, a possible mastectomy, my whole self to Him.

I noticed something Saturday night while sitting with Lee at the movies. We were sitting extra close, in the back seat of our friends' car, part of us touching. It was as though we were drawing strength from each other. I liked the feeling. Through the years we had grown out of the habit of exchanging affectionate gestures such as holding hands or a warm pat on the behind. Little by little these small but meaningful gestures were recurring.

Sunday morning I taught the freshman girls' Sunday School class. It was an emotional experience to share my cancer story with those lovable girls, Candy's friends. I was so caught up in reliving those memorable days that our class was still in session some time after the church service had begun. When I slipped into my place beside Lee I noticed some sympathetic glances directed our way. It looked as if word had gotten out that Janie had another undetermined lump. The lady to my left gave me a knowing hug and, as I squeezed past her to my seat, whispered, "We're praying for you." It suddenly occured to me that *she* had had a double mastectomy! I made a mental note to ask Dr. Allen about the possibility of his giving me two silicone implants while I was under anesthetic if the prognosis on Tuesday required another mastectomy. Following the worship service, several members expressed concern while others appeared uncomfortable and to be avoiding me. I understood.

Monday dawned clear with a pale November sun illuminating the landscape. A tennis date with Marion at the clay courts by lovely Lake Ellyn helped prepare me physically and emotionally to enter the hospital for lab work later that afternoon: a chest X-ray, a blood sample, and an EKG. During the cardiogram I was asked to lie back on a black leather contour chair, bare from the waist up. I must admit that the appearance of my remaining left breast was conspicuous without its mate and I considered it with fond affection. Who knows? It might no longer be a part of me by the weekend. For years I had viewed it and its twin as undersized and less than beautiful. This day it looked positively ravishing.

I was told to report to the hospital at 6:30 the next morning for surgery. Surgical patients were requested to remove all makeup, nail polish, and wigs, and to eat or drink nothing after midnight, not even a sip of water. This included the brushing of teeth.

Tuesday night I slept well in spite of the fact that Scott joined us in our bed complaining of leg cramps. I awakened famished, as usual, and tried to ignore the aroma of fresh toast Lee was enjoying in the kitchen. Instead, I shampooed and curled my hair and set my spirit in tune with God. During the brief drive to the hospital I remember hearing Eddy Arnold sing, "Have I Told You Lately That I Love You" and I thought of my sister Mary, his number one fan.

My hospital stay was to be short-term, perhaps seven or

eight hours overall. Two nurses wearing big smiles accompanied me to a pre-op ladies' dressing room where I was handed a pale blue gown, a striped robe, and slippers. Wearing my new uniform, I joined Lee in a pre-op waiting room. It had one other occupant, a gray-haired woman, dressed identically to me. Marks from her knee-length hose showed below her striped robe. Lee and I sat side by side, shoulders, arms, and legs touching. Although we didn't have much to say, the feelings between us were close and companionable. As he sketched landscaping plans, I checked the daily reading in *Streams in the Desert* which I had slipped into my purse. The Scripture verse read: *"That the power of Christ may rest upon me"* (2 Cor. 12:9). The meditation made the point that God allowed Jacob's crisis to close around him and bring him to the place where he could take hold of God as he otherwise never would have done. From that perilous experience, Jacob matured in his faith and knowledge of God, and in the power of a new and victorious life.

I reacted to these statements with a positive attitude. Apparently, God wasn't through testing my faith. He must want me to learn more of His power and peace in a time of crisis. I was learning to live moment by moment from the center out, rather than from the outside in. I reminded myself that the Presence of God lived *within me!*

It wasn't long before a white-clad figure came for me. I inhaled the scent of Jovan's Sex Appeal as I kissed Lee goodbye. Gosh, after twenty-four years of marriage his kisses still tasted good. For what must have been the tenth time I was asked whether I had had anything to eat or drink and whether I was allergic to any drugs. I was wheeled for the third time in a year into an operating room of the Central DuPage Hospital. When the favorite figure of Dr. Allen entered, I joshed, "Tell the truth, you just came from playing a set or two at the Racket Club. Right?" Imagine my surprise when he nodded a yes to me. "That's not fair," I continued,

"I can't play until tomorrow. I *can* play tomorrow, can't I?"

"You can." (A man of few words. He doesn't need words.)

I asked him if he would give me two new silicone breasts, augmentation, if it turned out that I needed a second mastectomy. And, please, could I have the reconstruction while I was still under the anesthetic?

"That sounds like a great idea."

With that reassurance I remember commenting that I was growing sleepy and they hadn't given me a mask to sniff. The smiling anesthesiologist (everyone smiled in this hospital) explained that he had given me a needle of sodium pentathol while I was chatting with Dr. Allen. I consciously relinquished myself to God and to His competent surgeon for whom I had enormous affection.

The next thing I remember was the sound of Lee's happy voice, "Honey, he removed the lump and it appears to be free of cancer! Dr. Allen decided not to do a frozen section, he was so sure." I recall feeling immense joy and then sleep took over again. Later, Lee explained he'd been told that the lump and some surrounding tissue had been sent to the pathology lab for seventy-two hours of testing.

After a couple of hours I roused enough to realize that I needed to use the bathroom. Whatever from? (Not even a sip of water.) Then I noticed the I.V. dripping into my left arm. It came back to me that in the operating room I had asked that they not put the I.V. into my right arm. It seems this is not a wise procedure when the breast and lymph nodes have been removed. After I'd used the bathroom, the nurse suggested that I try to sit up out in the pre-op waiting room. I murmured that I would much rather lie down and go back to sleep. When she explained that a surgical patient must be in an upright position for at least one half-hour before being permitted to go home, I permitted her to prop me up in a chair with pillows and a blanket. Through half-closed eyes I noticed at least two other patients in the same drowsy position and that, of all things, there was a TV soap opera bouncing into the room—*The Doctors*. Would you believe that a doctor was performing surgery and at the same time was admonishing his nurse, "Catch that bleeder! This thing isn't going right at all. Nurse! Help me stop the bleeding!" I glanced from the TV screen to a patient who obviously hadn't been to the operating room yet (her eyes were all the way open and her hair was immaculate) and said, "This isn't exactly the best thing for you to be watching, is it?" She agreed, but neither one of us was able to reach the on-off button and there was not a nurse in sight. Those of us who had had surgery were having enough trouble trying to remain upright. All I could envision was our comfortable bed with its new brown blanket which Lee and I had made up together earlier that morning.

It was a comical scene. We resembled a select group of blue-and-white-striped sleepwalkers. A pretty young girl, who had also had a breast biopsy, was obviously uncomfortable. Her husband, wearing a blue knit cap and blue tattoos, appeared detached and unsympathetic. I suggested that he come over and sit next to his hurting wife, and in the meantime I groggily pulled up my feet to make room for him. There was no response; he remained detached and indifferent. Tears were making tracks down her cheeks when a smiling nurse appeared to ask if everything was satisfactory. I nodded a no in the direction of the young woman. Her complaint of pain in the area of her incision suddenly made me aware that I had a similar pain but had been too absorbed in my Good News Report to be conscious of it. The nurse encouraged me to get dressed and then scolded me for not accepting her help. I heard Dr. Allen being paged and learned they were trying to locate him for a pain pill prescription for me. In no time the nurse at the desk called Lee at home to come get me. It was 2:30 P.M. on the face of our bedside radio when I returned to slumberland.

22

A Lot to Be Thankful For

Around 5:30 P.M. I awakened, refreshed and free from any discomfort, to the muted sounds of children. One by one they stopped by our bedroom. Kim was off to an away volleyball game. Candy, just in from basketball practice, expressed interest in attending Kim's game. Lee, too, wanted to see Kim play. Scott added, "Me too." And I thought, wow, they really take a radical recovery for granted around here.

Lee suggested to Scott that he stay home with Mom, but Scott wanted to go to the game. I decided not to feel sorry for myself and said they all should go. I would be fine. But would they please first go down and warm up the chili I had planned for supper. Then Lee anounced firmly that Scott would remain at home to take care of Mom. Scott concurred. The phone rang and it was Luci who, when she learned what the menu was to be, insisted on bringing over something more appropriate for the recovering-from-anesthetic patient. My visiting angel appeared in the doorway a short time later bearing gifts of affection, salad, and roast beef sandwiches. Scott and I snuggled the evening away in the super-sized bed, my eyes shut, my body slackened with sleep. I adored the company of my nine-year-old male nurse.

Much later I discovered the following statement in Scott's

132

"Do For Others" book for Sunday School: "I stayed home with my Mom. But I wanted to go to the volleyball game." I looked closely, and noticed that he had crossed out the second sentence. Perhaps the evening had turned out to be more satisfying than sacrificial.

The expressions on the faces of my tennis companions contained a mixture of surprise and something I couldn't define as I rushed into the Racket Club the next day. The team captain announced that I would be playing first with Gib as my partner. During the first three or four games I took deep breaths and determined to put mind (relaxed, controlled strokes) over matter (I was just out of surgery and still feeling shaky). The power of positive thinking won. We took the first set 6-3; the second 6-0. The time totaled forty minutes.

The next afternoon Luci and I decided to ride horseback. The horses seemed unusually spirited in the gray November air, and we exclaimed at the bleak beauty of the countryside. Just before crossing the river a pack of red-tailed hawks swooped overhead to pause motionless in the frozen air. It seemed as though they were appraising us. Muted shades of beige and brown stretched endlessly everywhere. Dried weeds and bare-leafed branches shivered in the wind and we had to kick our horses into a canter to keep warm. I was alive with the joy of a good report from Dr. Allen and the familiar rhythm of riding horseback and being with a special friend, one who responded to the lovely landscape as I did. We arrived back at the stable with skin tingling and souls refreshed by God's paintbrush.

By the weekend I began to experience soreness and occasional stabbing pains in my stitches. I chose to ignore them. I couldn't. Monday night I had severe muscular spasms in my left breast. Only when I remained perfectly still, flat on my back, did they stop. Even a slight motion sideways or towards a sitting position resulted in extreme pain, and I screamed with surprise as they occurred again and again. Lee stood patiently in our bedroom with a sleeping pill and

glass of water while I struggled to find a position in which I
could swallow. We discussed what could have contributed to
this severe discomfort. That day I had played one and a-half
hours of tennis. Could this be it? After being home from the
hospital nearly a week I found that if I remained flat on my
back at night the pains disappeared. Since I was a tummy
sleeper, this was an awkward adjustment. Second choice was
sleeping on my side. However, when I tentatively tried to
turn to one side I was met with intense pain. Tuesday morning I reluctantly turned down a tennis invitation. Instead, I
washed windows all morning. They glistened in the afternoon sunshine. Tuesday night the pains were worse. When I
removed my bra getting ready for bed my entire breast
began to throb and I climbed into bed like a hundred-year-
old woman crippled with arthritis. Only this time I swal-
lowed a pain pill and added a sleeping pill at a safe interval.

Wednesday morning, the day before Thanksgiving, Dr.
Allen was to remove the stitches. Entering the examining
room, he said, "You've been suffering, haven't you?" I dis-
solved in tears. How could he have known?

"Have you been playing too much tennis?" he gently
inquired.

"Yes." Meekly.

He explained that he had done more than remove the
lump, and he was not surprised that I was having a lot of
pain at this point. In removing surrounding tissue he had
had to suture several layers and pull skin across a sort of cre-
vice. This was all trying to heal, nerves had been cut, and
the pain was a natural result of the procedure. As he reached
out and gently touched the area, I winced. He suggested
that we wait another week before removing the six black
stitches. I could play as much tennis as I wanted; it could not
damage anything. However, he warned, I would suffer discomfort in proportion to how active I had been that particular day. He gave me another prescription for pain and we
parted.

Preparing for a Thanksgiving dinner for two families, ours and Bob and Marion's, twelve of us in all, left little time for inactivity that afternoon. Nevertheless, that did not prevent me from sharing an outpouring of thankfulness with the members of our church family at our traditional Thanksgiving morning service of praise. In a clear, quiet voice I thanked Him for returning the spark to long and lonely years in our marriage, for the friendship of Bob and Marion's family, and for the fact that I was free of cancer after a recent lumpectomy. People came by to hug me after the service. I wasn't sure why. All I knew was that I felt close to them and that I was very, very happy. We drove to our home in the country and enjoyed a nearly perfect day that will linger long in memory.

#

Straight Talk: Breast Reconstruction, Prostheses, Prevention, and Recovery Aids

BREAST RECONSTRUCTION

My surgeon discussed the possibility of breast reconstruction with me both before and after surgery. He felt that I was an ideal candidate for reconstruction. Since my lump was small and located on the lower outside of my breast, he was able to leave a fair amount of skin covering the chest wall, as well as the areola, the reddish, pigmented circle surrounding the nipple.

I Am Whole Again by Jean Zalon pleads the case for breast reconstruction after mastectomy and holds out new hope to every woman who has ever had breast surgery—as well as every woman who has ever feared it. I found the book a moving, inspiring story.

In 1970 Jean Zalon underwent a radical mastectomy. In *I Am Whole Again* she describes the severe emotional trauma she suffered afterward and her search for a surgeon to reconstruct her breast. She reports that when she was finally able to look at her body with pleasure, she felt "not just reconstructed but reborn."

Ms. Zalon not only prepares women for what to expect but advises how to seek the best help, how to deal with family and friends, exactly what surgical procedures are involved.

To help readers understand how breast loss affects women, especially in a society where the female breast is so intimately associated with a woman's sexuality and self-esteem, she relates her conversations with several women who have also undergone mastectomies.

The following information regarding reconstruction has been derived in part from this informative, helpful book.

The most widely performed reconstruction involves the creation of a pocket under the skin and the insertion of an implant shaped like a breast. The implant is a silicone gel contained in a pliable plastic bag. The implants most generally used come in a number of sizes, but the choice of size is less related to the dimensions of the original breast than to the amount of skin available to form a cover over the insert. Sometimes only a very small implant can be used at the beginning. Then later, when the skin stretches out a bit, the incision can be reopened and a larger mound placed in the pocket.

Depending on the surgeon who performs the operation, the incision for the implant may be vertical or horizontal. The horizontal incision usually coincides with the natural skin fold under the breast and is therefore not very noticeable. The vertical scar is slightly visible.

The patient who is satisfied to regain a sense of wholeness, recapture some degree of cleavage and look reasonably presentable in a bra may be able to ignore either minor or major imbalance that often results from left to right, since the reconstructed breast will not always match the healthy remaining one.

Studies show that the artificial breast does not interfere with either manual or X-ray examinations. And surgeons now are doing fewer radical mastectomies which involve the removal of the breast, underlying tissue and muscle, and surrounding tissue. With the more moderate operations (simple, modified, or subcutaneous mastectomies) surgeons leave the chest wall muscle, which can then be used to anchor the artificial breast. While the appearance of a patient cannot be restored to that before surgery, breast reconstruction does offer a great deal to the patient, enabling her both to look and to feel more like a woman. Breasts are cherished by women as a badge of motherhood, as a sign of femininity, and as an important psycho-sexual symbol.

Frequently the nipple can be spared and in some cases an artificial nipple can be made from other tissue. In most cases today, the nipple and areola are created from labial tissue from around the vagina. A reconstructed nipple is not erectile and lacks sensitivity to sexual stimulation. This is unavoidable, since the mammary nerves were removed in the mastectomy and the new nipple's only connection is to the skin around it.

At this writing it has been five years since my mastectomy and I am considering breast reconstruction. Why, you might ask?

(1) Both my surgeon and oncologist have assured me that in my case it would be an uncomplicated, uplifting operation.

(2) I would feel secure in my scoop-necked tennis dresses and swimsuits.

(3) When undressed I would feel more balanced, attractive, and womanly. For Lee and me, our sex life is becoming an increasingly more important part of our relationship. We find nudity both sensuous and stimulating.

PROSTHESES

Since I was considering reconstruction, I was not anxious to invest $100 in a breast form. In the meantime, I used a variety of stuffing to fill out the right cup of my bras, such as large wads of cotton or a pair of nylon hose, and I pinned a tennis sock into my swim suit.

In response to my question as to how soon I could play tennis after breast reconstruction, Dr. Allen said approximately five weeks for a hard-hitting tennis player. This described my game. It was March when I was able to resume play after my mastectomy. Soon it would be summer and the tournament tennis season would be upon us. I decided that the fast-approaching tennis season held greater appeal for me than a new breast.

With this decision it was time to replace my cotton-stuffed bra with a prosthesis. My friend Gretchen, who had recently had a mastectomy, told me that she had purchased a weighted, fluid-filled, natural-contoured prosthesis right in Wheaton.

One day, soon after our phone conversation, we met unexpectedly at an indoor Racket Club where I was to substitute in a weekly group of tennis players. Before we went out on the courts I approached Gretchen in the locker room and whispered, "Say, how would you like to swap the contents of our bras? Would you let me try your new prosthesis?"

"Sure," she responded immediately.

In a jiffy she reached inside her tennis dress and handed me a soft, flesh-colored breast form complete with its own nipple, while I removed my graying wad of cotton for her bra. I glanced around to see whether we had been observed while making the exchange, at the same time admiring Gretchen's unself-consciousness.

It seemed like only yesterday (it had been over two months) I had answered the phone one afternoon to hear Gretchen sob, "Janie, I need some information. I just discovered a lump in my left breast." My immediate thought was, "It's good it's her *left* breast. A mastectomy won't interfere with her tennis game." (My only contact with Gretchen had been on the tennis court.) Now here she was as attractive as ever, her pale blond hair framing a Dresden-doll face. There was a twinkle in her blue eyes as she hurried out onto the courts calling, "See how you like it. Meet you back here after tennis."

I was anxious to notice whether my new breast would ride

up when I raised my arm to serve. It didn't! After only a few sets I began to feel at home with my visiting tenant. Tucked inside the right cup of my bra, it adhered to my skin nicely, and I was hardly conscious of its presence. Gretchen was playing two courts away. "It's neat!" I shouted to her, making the appropriate sign with curled right thumb and forefinger. She grinned her response and I couldn't help thinking, "If these girls only knew . . ."

Later we giggled in the locker room as we again made the exchange. I noted that my wad of cotton was soaking wet whereas the breast form wasn't.

The very next day I visited the shop in Wheaton that sells everything for the mastectomy patient. I tried on a variety of types of breast forms before making my final decision to one like Gretchen's. (Only I needed a size larger. I hate braggers.) Since then I have purchased a mastectomy swimsuit from this same shop. The suit appears like any other except that it comes with a hidden inside pocket in which to slide one's prosthesis. The owner of the shop had had a mastectomy, and consequently she is both aware of and sensitive to her customers' needs. The shop reeks of good taste and is supplied with an enchanting variety of garments such as evening gowns, lingerie, bras, swimsuits, etc., tailored for the mastectomy patient. It also boasts spacious dressing rooms with upholstered chairs and three-way mirrors where the shopper is guaranteed maximum privacy.

I was careful to place my breast form in the same location each evening when undressing for bed. It would be terrible to lose such a valuable and costly item. Well, one July day the inevitable happened. I reached into my clothes closet to discover it MISSING. After a thorough search it was STILL MISSING. I mentally retraced my steps. I finally remembered I had changed at the club from my swimsuit into a strappy summer dress before going for a doctor's checkup. Since that particular dress required my black strapless padded bra, I had no need to wear my close companion, my prosthesis.

Perhaps one of the lifeguards found it either in the shower or the dressing room. But would she recognize it as an artificial breast? I forced myself to call the club and spoke to the owner's wife who said she would check and call me right back. I waited—my heart in my mouth.

"I can't find it, Janie, but I'll talk to each of the life guards and see if anyone has seen it. Would you mind if I make a suggestion?" she chortled. "Why don't you count before leaving next time?"

I forced a laugh.

The next twelve hours dragged by.

The next afternoon I drove reluctantly to the smart shop where I had purchased my form and its charming owner *loaned* me a new one. As soon as I reached home my mother-in-law announced, "You are supposed to call the club." My heart raced. ,

"Janie," Leslie's calm voice said, "it seems that my daughter found your prosthesis in one of the shower dressing rooms, placed it in a brown paper bag, and put it on a shelf under the front desk. She failed to mention this to me or to anyone else."

I hastily returned my borrowed form and retrieved my trusty companion at the club—vowing never to let it out of my sight again.

PREVENTION

Current statistics are that fourteen out of every fifteen women will never get breast cancer. However, every woman needs to guard against the disease with regular physical examinations and a monthly breast self-examination. When breast cancer is found early, before it has spread, the chances of cure are very high. ALL CHANGES—lumps, nipple discharge, unusual sensation or other breast change—should always receive prompt, expert medical examination.

Bathing or showering is your moment to take care of yourself, to take time for a breast self-examination. As you wash, while your skin is slippery, it's a simple thing to do. Keep your fingers flat and touch every part of each breast. Feel gently for a lump or thickening. Why? Because it could save your life. After your shower, take a moment for a more thorough check.

Monthly self-examination helps a woman know the normal consistency of her breasts, enabling her to identify any change.

Ninety-five percent of all breast cancers are discovered by women themselves.

Despite the fact that a high percentage of breast lumps will prove to be harmless, it is important to see your physician as soon as possible if you discover a lump or thickening.

Breast cancer is highly curable. The odds are in your favor and they'll improve, if you act on what you know right now.

The above information has been taken from a small pamphlet put out by the American Cancer Society.

The February 15, 1976, issue of *Modern People* carried a number of interesting findings on the relation of cancer and stress. There exists the possibility that cancer may in some few cases be psychosomatic. Cancer researchers working at Johns Hopkins University are finding increasing indications that cancer is mental, or that cancer can be triggered by mental or emotional causes.

V. R. Riley of the Northwest Research Foundation in Seattle, Washington, found that the crucial factor in the development of cancers was stress. He completed some astounding laboratory experiments in that regard on mice.

Many researchers have observed the same thing where people are concerned. Naturally, some of us are able to handle stress and don't develop cancers. But many people cannot.

The connection between emotions and cancer has been talked about for over a generation now. In his book *No Mira-*

cles Among Friends, written in the '50s, a British surgeon, Sir Heneg Ogilvie, said: "The happy man never gets cancer." Of course, what makes one person happy, might make another unhappy. But his point was this: It now seems almost certain that if something in your life changes to make you much less happy or permanently unhappy, you are a prime candidate for cancer. And, if you can keep in your life that which makes you basically happy, you are going a long way toward protecting yourself against cancer.

One thing seems sure—mental state is crucial in dealing with cancer.

The same issue of *Modern People* mentioned above also stated that the National Institute of Cancer in Milan, Italy, is working on a report called "Toward An Understanding of Cancer as a Psychosomatic Phenomenon." The main author of the study, Dr. Filippo Beringheli, was said to be a prime candidate for the Nobel Prize.

Greece is working on a similar study. At the University of Athens, Dr. N. C. Rassidakis has shown cancer, diabetes, and schizophrenia all to be linked by a strong mental factor. One of the proofs for this is "the frequent appearance of these diseases when there is the greatest mental turmoil" together with "the disappearance of anxiety once the disease is established."

AIDS FOR RECOVERY

Lee was far more concerned about my recovery than he let on. The fact that he suffered two heart attacks, fortunately mild ones, six weeks after my surgery confirmed this supposition. His ready grin and frequent wisecracks were covering a mask of concern. I want to emphasize, however, that from the day the lump was discovered and throughout my confinement and recuperation, he was attentive, loving, and managed to keep a light touch.

Our marriage relationship was strengthened by Lee's obvious acceptance of the loss of my breast. His manner did not suggest that I was any less of a woman or less attractive because I was flat on one side. Instead, we both were excited that Dr. Allen was certain he had removed all of the cancer and I was going to be around for a long time. How very fortunate I was, we both agreed, that the cancer had not spread to the lymph nodes. My chances for a complete recovery were excellent.

I am thankful that the series of events the six days I spent in the hospital did not allow time to think about the state of our marriage; that kind of stress, as already noted, could have had a very negative effect. Instead, each day was one of unusual optimism and expectancy. I was in the middle of an adventure with God as my Guide. My thoughts upon waking were: What good thing are we going to do together today, Lord? I had entrusted myself, my present, my future, my whole life, to Him, and He and I *together* were going to make things happen. My mental state was so positive and accepting that there was little room for negative thoughts such as death, pain, distrust, disfigurement, failure.

I believe that my quick mobility so soon after my mastectomy was unusual. Looking back, I can point to several contributing factors. For one thing, my sports-oriented lifestyle and love of the outdoors had kept me in top physical condition. My earliest memories are of the outdoors. My mother, an avid nature lover, saw to it that as babies and young children we were in the open air whenever possible. All of us were born in summer, and we took our naps in a baby buggy covered with mosquito netting, near the flower garden. We shared in a childhood where playing baseball in the cow pasture and developing skill with a slingshot were considered the norm. Second, from both of our parents we inherited not only a strong love of tennis, but a fierce spirit of competitiveness. Additional determination to excel resulted from our parents' expectations of us as model children of the respected pastor of a mainline Philadelphia Presbyterian Church. Third, in spite of the fact that my marriage wasn't all that it should be, I loved life and was anxious to return to the world of ordinary people and to get on with the business of living and loving. Friends have used the words *vivacious, intense, alive,* and *exuberant* to describe me. I've had that positive attitude toward life ever since I can remember.

Another aid for recovery is the Reach to Recovery program. In many hospitals this is the only counseling that is offered. The visit I had from Barbara (described in chapter 15) was typical. A cheerful, outgoing volunteer who has already undergone a mastectomy herself comes to visit you. She explains a series of exercises to promote physical rehabilitation and also shows you various prosthetic forms designed to go inside the bra. This is a terrific morale-builder. I had supplemented the Reach to Recovery exercises by throwing a tennis ball against the wall at the hospital.

The chief thrust of Reach to Recovery, the brilliant inspiration of its founder, Terese Lasser, is to remind the mastectomy patient that she is not alone. This indispensable service is the turning point for many women in their recovery.

ENCORE, the YWCA Post-Mastectomy Group Rehabilitation Program, is another valuable aid for a faster recovery. ENCORE is a special exercise and discussion program developed by a woman who has recovered from a mastectomy herself—Helen Glines Kohut, R.N. Besides being a registered nurse, Mrs. Kohut is also a qualified instructor of swimming and ballet.

The ENCORE program, developed in 1972, for the most part does achieve the physical and psychological goals it sets, in short, to help women feel whole again. ENCORE sessions are held once a week and are about an hour and a half long. Each session is divided into three parts—floor exercises, pool exercises, and class discussions. The floor exercises are gentle ones done to music. They are designed to tone and strengthen the affected arm as a part of total body fitness.

Part of the session is devoted to sharing your experiences or airing your troubles, and there is a chance to share joy and laughter, too.

Another portion of each session is spent in the pool. Water therapy is one of the quickest ways to redevelop muscles and regain flexibility.

In a recent conversation I had with Dr. Baker, I asked him if he could confirm a suspicion of mine. "Is it not true that the strongest enemies of cancer are a strong, positive attitude towards all aspects of life and the endeavor to keep stress at a minimum?"

"Yes," he agreed, "but be sure to mention that genetics and environment are also contributing factors."

Of all the sources I checked for helpful material on cancer, my favorite is *Getting Well Again: A Step-by-Step, Self-Help Guide to Overcoming Cancer for Patients and Their Families* by Dr. Carl Symington and Stephanie Matthews-Symington. The dust cover of the book beautifully describes what it has to offer, and the content lives up to the expectations that are generated.

> In this book, Dr. Carl Symington and Stephanie Matthews-Symington, leading practitioners in the field of the psychological causes and treatment of cancer, describe how patients can apply *on their own* the potentially life-saving and life-extending procedures they have developed at their world-famous treatment center in Fort Worth, Texas.
>
> The psychological techniques that the Symingtons recommend *do not replace* standard medical procedures, but are used *in conjunction with* them. The objective is to help patients help themselves by creating the best environment—internally and externally—for their own recovery.
>
> Specifically, *Getting Well Again* describes how an individual's reaction to stress and other emotional factors may have contributed to the onset and progress (or recurrence) of the disease and gives detailed instructions to help patients recognize and deal with these elements in their lives.

Using the experiences of hundreds of patients with whom they have worked in Fort Worth, the Symingtons show how their treatment program—which includes techniques for learning positive attitudes, relaxation, visualization, goal-setting, managing pain, exercising and building an "emotional support system"—will not only enhance patients' chances for recovery but will substantially improve the quality of life.

The authors give the "will to live" a scientific basis and demonstrate how positive expectancies and a habit of psychological self-awareness and self-care can play a significant role for anyone in maintaining health, and for the cancer patient in getting well again.

The authors say:

There is a clear link between stress and illness, a link so strong that it is possible to predict illness based on the amount of stress in people's lives. . . .

For instance, physicians have observed that illness is more likely to occur following highly stressful events in people's lives. Many doctors have noticed that when their patients suffered major emotional upsets, there was an increase not only in diseases usually acknowledged to be susceptible to emotional influences—ulcers, high blood pressure, heart disease, headaches—but also in infectious diseases, backaches, and even accidents. . . . Stress may accumulate to the point that the individual simply can no longer cope and consequently becomes ill.

The Symingtons have done much to educate people about the role patients can play in overcoming cancer and to encourage them to accept responsibility for their disease, accept responsibility for healing, and to learn about the techniques for unlocking powers that can be found within themselves.

Coupled with the resources of a strong spiritual faith, and the loving support of family and friends, the Symingtons' book can be invaluable to cancer sufferers. And it could very well help many people avoid cancer altogether.

Caribbean Vacation

January 28, 1979

Today is the anniversary of my first biopsy—the day Dr. Allen discovered a suspicious-looking lump that was confirmed to be cancer. It hardly seems possible that Lee and I are on a plane returning from twelve delicious days of vacation in the Caribbean.

With great care Lee planned that we spend five days each on two separate islands. Of primary importance to him was that we be where there were a minimum of tourists, unspoiled tropical beauty, and consistently warm temperatures. He succeeded. One subzero day he announced that we had reservations to fly to the island of Tortola on Monday, January 16.

As a result of his careful planning we enjoyed perfect relaxation from the stress and demands of everyday pressures. Shedding children, inhibitions, and clothes I gradually unwound and became fully aware of my identity as a woman, wife, and lover. Together we discovered the primitive beauty of the capital of the British Virgin Islands. Each day the hotel where we stayed provided a land rover which transported us to snowy white secluded beaches where we snorkled, plunged through breakers and lay in the sunlight on bright beaches below the cloud-hung green wall of the mountains. In the late afternoons, salty and sun-soaked, we returned to the privacy of our room with the bamboo swing. The fact that I had one breast was unimportant. The fact that we were alive and in love again was.

We made genuine friends with Peter and Mary, the hotel manager and his wife, and several other guests. With them we explored this largely undiscovered island with its rugged mountains, lush vegetation and crystal clear aquamarine sea. I used large sunglasses to hide my tears the morning we bid farewell to the cluster of close companions we had grown to love.

Our tiny plane set down on the island of St. Maarten, population one thousand, which is entirely different from any other place in the world. We stayed at a place on a mile-long private beach, where our room, the dining area, and the terrace all provided a spectacular view of the ocean. After discovering several chaise lounges within a short distance from our room on the ground floor, on two mornings we transferred our sleepy selves to watch the sun rise slowly over the sparkling sea. There was ample time for beneath-the-surface conversation, thinking long thoughts, re-evaluating our priorities, and spontaneous touching. It was a chance to rediscover each other; what had lain unspoken surfaced and resulted in affection and affirmation. For the first time in a long time there was nothing separating us. Every word went to the heart with an ease I could not believe. We talked and talked, but the thing we both understood did not need to be said.

One day we joined another couple and explored the island, stopping to admire romantic coasts with inlets, bays, beaches, and mountainous countryside. Lush hills, valleys, and pastures were dotted with goats. The picture was one of West Indian beauty, of quaint villages and friendly people. One of our stops included a cool coconut drink and our first encounter with escargots—snails. A wild yellow canary joined us and Carol and Larry, our new friends, as we stabbed the slippery contents of the shells and dipped them in tangy sauce.

We arrived back in Chicago bronzed by the sun, richer in relationship, and refreshed in spirit. Other valuables included a wealth of mellow memories and a determination to live fully in the now. Priorities and values came into focus—such as being in right relationship with God, the value of hard work, exercising one's God given talents, the importance of contentment, and the necessity of love and laughter.

We were greeted at O'Hare airport by our children in a swirling snowstorm and began to live the first day of the rest of our lives.

25

When We're Too Busy—by Lee

As Janie and I attempted to put our marriage back together we encountered several roadblocks.

One of the most difficult areas to handle was the paradox in several things that occurred in the church. I experienced situations where one thing was said, yet another was practiced. I discovered that "admitted failure does not necessarily result in practiced forgiveness."

For years, professionals and leaders in the church design programs, plan worship services, and arrange faith-challenging retreat weekends to encourage the child of God to be honest, vulnerable, and sensitive. Then, I found, when a person becomes honest and admits imperfection, that action-step by the confessor becomes an isolation-step for him as well.

In several instances, the committees, retreats, study groups and even the prayers in public places proved to be words—not actions, not a way of life.

We, the church, talk about having found real hope, about caring for one another. We demand integrity in wanting to share this kind of life with others outside of the Church. We invest much time studying the forgiveness that God gives and discussing the redemptive qualities of the Church. However, when the opportunities arrive to express these qualities we often find ourselves too busy to become involved.

I look back now and remember that following a church service people heading towards me would quickly turn and head in the other direction. I remember walking down the aisle in the grocery store and watching fellow church members turn and navigate their shopping carts in the opposite direction. (I must admit that on one occasion—or maybe it was more than once—I intentionally headed my cart for their "escape route" so that we would be forced to meet and speak.)

Imagine—these are representatives of God's family. We're supposed to be the caring and sensitive ones of this world. We are ambassadors that God has sent and we can't be sensitive enough to care for one another. What is going to make us care for those unappealing and failing ones out in the world where we live and walk from day to day?

My relationship with my wife was made more difficult because of the rejection that occurred for me and my family members. During these three struggling years after my Jamaican experience I received numerous phone calls from people in the church, asking to see me in private. I listened as men and women, with hearts broken and lives weighed down with guilt, poured out their failures and sins with tears and groanings that I too, had experienced. One by one, I listened to them, prayed and cried with them and expressed caring. Over and over I heard them say, "Don't tell anyone. Please don't tell the Church; they would never understand."

Many times I questioned why I had allowed myself to go through the anguish of asking forgiveness of my church and making myself vulnerable. What good would it all do? As time has passed, I've found that with a broken heart and buckets of tears I was more able to respond to people who were buried in guilt and pain and to love them. A wounded man is able to respond to a wounded man; a failure is able to respond to a failure; a sinner is able to respond to a sinner—these were lines I had read or heard many times. But when I needed a wounded listener . . . I struggled to find one. I saw all kinds of "perfect people." I saw all kinds of beautiful people leading committees and retreats and youth groups. I saw "sinners saved by grace," but all I needed was a sinner who cared enough to listen, to respond in a caring way, and to love me for who I was.

The more I study the Word, the more I see this kind of compassion in the life of Jesus. Jesus was in the "people business," and that's where I feel God has called each of us. If we're too busy to honestly, sensitively, and singularly listen to another wounded person, we're too busy. I mean too busy in church business. Too busy meeting committee responsibilities. Too busy teaching Sunday School about God's love. Too busy having the ideal worship service. Too busy going to Bible study. Too busy at board meetings. Too busy serving God. Too busy preaching love and forgiveness. Too busy to see and respond to needy people across this land and the world.

Maybe we are all too busy.

As I write this my heart becomes extremely heavy and sad, because *I* was too busy talking—too busy to listen.

I want to be different than I was. My daily prayer is that God will grant me the sense and sensitivity to know when and where to be—and when and where to listen, to love, and not to judge.

During the past year Steve, our oldest boy, and I have shared many long hours of talking and listening to each other. I've learned so much from my own son. His sensitive loving spirit has touched my heart and life. I long to be the man and father he has encouraged me to be.

Today, when Janie and I consider all the people that God has directed into our lives, we feel truly blessed. I used to consider many things as signs or symbols of success. Now I feel that if people could say of me, my wife, and my

children, "That family really *cares for people,*" I would feel
that we're doing what God wants us to do, and be. *The
Living Bible* reads in 1 John 3:18: "Let us stop just saying
we love people; let us really love them, and show it by our
actions."

26

Listening to the Signals

The phone call that interrupted my universe shortly after Lee's return from Jamaica in 1974 almost destroyed me. The pain that followed was unbearable as I felt betrayed by two of the people closest to me. Hours, days, months, of agony followed. I asked God for a forgiving spirit. It did not come. I read David Augsburger's book and others on the importance of forgiveness; it loomed an impossible task. My hurt seemed too deep for healing.

That was the fall I accepted the position of secretary of the English Department at Wheaton College. As it was the largest department on campus, my job kept me too busy to have time to think.

As repressed negative emotions took their toll, I became vulnerable to cancer, the hated monster that had visited my sister, mother and grandmother. My body's natural resistance to disease was down. The cancer in my marriage finally contributed to a cancer in my body. There is a popular concept that much disease occurs when we have a lowered resistance. This comes about when we disregard God's natural laws by working harder than He intends us to do. It also occurs when we are under emotional stress. By working eight hours four days each week and attempting to maintain a clean, well-executed home, and be an attentive, supportive parent I was placing myself under pressure. It was important to me and to the girls that I show up at their volleyball, basketball, softball, and tennis games. My schedule overflowed with responsibilities. And in addition to all of this I was making a supreme attempt to forgive and forget my husband's failings.

The inevitable happened. I became impatient and discouraged. Pressure and frustration multiplied. I found myself crying without any warning. When watching a romantic movie I would suddenly dissolve in tears. My heart ached. My imagination wandered. It hurt to be around happy couples. The combination of anxiety, uncertainty, hating, and hurting made me vulnerable to disease.

In an article in *New Woman* magazine the authors stated that a bad relationship is as destructive to good health as the lack of an essential nutrient. For people living with each other to remain in healthy relationship, it takes work, dedication and open communication. Without communication no real relationship is possible.

The article, "The Essential Ingredients in Being Well," went on to say that the will to be well is present in everyone, but feelings like fear, resentment and despair may cloud the relationship you have with your inner wisdom. Tension and fatigue may also set up a barrier which prevents some of your maintenance and surveillance mechanisms from operating.

Whether you are healthy or ill depends on a vital balance, the authors tell us. Recovery from an illness has more to do with a healthy attitude than with the intervention of outside forces such as doctors, drugs or healers. In fact, the whole fabric of health is directly tied into the daily operation of the will to be well. Attempt more and more to do those things which bring on a feeling of well being.

Growth is an essential ingredient in aliveness. If you reach a certain level in living and then stop, you will begin to stagnate, to grow dull. Ask yourself if you are spending your time and energy the way you want to be spending them. What are your priorities, both short and long range? It pays to be clear about what you want, and it even pays to be clear about what you don't want.

The article ended with this final, noteworthy statement. "I see clearly that my health depends largely on my attitudes, and that I can, and do, choose my attitude. I choose to be well."

Since I have had cancer I have devoured every article I have seen that relates to this dreaded disease. I am convinced that the number one cause of cancer is emotional stress. Recently I confronted an oncologist (cancer specialist) with this question and my suspicions were confirmed. Since that time I have taken active steps to promote the importance of excellent physical and emotional health.

People who live to a ripe age almost invariably do things they really enjoy doing, or just have a general sense of delight in the changing panorama of life.

In order to function fully and be able to face our problems squarely we need to get in touch with our own feelings. We need to become skilled to listen attentively to our own body's signals.

I believe my anger directed at Lee was a coverup for a bleak and bitter sense of personal failure. We had both failed as loving, responsible marriage partners. In my preoccupation with self-discovery and self-acceptance I neglected to meet needs of my husband. Eventually I ceased to become the object of Lee's desires. When reasons for heartbreak and distrust surfaced I became acquainted with disappointment and depression—and finally, disease. Because I had lived with the cancer in my marriage for so long, the cancer in my breast was not catastrophic for me. And since it was a small lump discovered in its earliest stages my doctor has good reason to believe that he got it all.

I trusted my earthly surgeon to remove the cancer in my breast. He did. Six months later I trusted my heavenly sur-

geon *to remove the cancer in my marriage. He did.* However, it wasn't until I truly believed that God could and would do this for me that He did. Mark 9:23 in the Living Bible tells me that anything is possible *if you have faith.* This promise is conditional. The final four words of this verse are significant. *Human nature says: Show me Lord, and I'll believe. God says: Believe, and I'll show you.* At long last I truly believed that my God could do even this for me. I *expected* God to act, and He did.

But O my soul, don't be discouraged. Don't be upset. Expect God to act! For I know that I shall again have plenty of reason to praise him for all that he will do. He is my help! He is my God! (Ps. 42:11).

27

A Prophecy Fulfilled

Do I still feel threatened by attractive women? Rarely. There are several possible explanations. Since jealousy has been my unwelcome companion most of my life, I give the credit to God's power to change me. Also, Lee is more sensitive to my feelings, now, and does not invite the attention of attractive women.

I have a sense of identity now. I like myself and feel loved and respected for who I am. Lee is Lee, and I am me. We are two individuals who bring to one another a greater degree of wholeness to share and enhance one another. Lee used to have certain expectations for me to achieve as wife, mother, and woman. He now allows me the freedom to be me. He now respects and loves the me who is truly me.

He has allowed God to make him more loving, less demanding. He no longer insists that I adjust to meet his needs. His quick defensive attitude has disappeared.

As predicted in the prophecy I was given by Rev. Winter, God has richly blessed our marriage and our household.

Since Lee and I got our marriage together, we have become a more effective tennis doubles team. It isn't that our individual games have improved. Rather, we have a new attitude of acceptance and affirmation of the other's skills. It had been our custom to compete in summer tournaments where we played in the A division. We noticed that the tension in our relationship peaked on the tennis court:

"Why does he have to destroy the ball all the time?"

"Not another double fault?"

"When is she going to move off the baseline and join me at the net?"

Thoughts like these kept interfering with our concentration and, consequently, our performance.

In the summer of 1979, Lee and I returned to the world of competition, played eleven tournament matches, and won all of them. There was a conspicuous lack of tension on the court—a result of the restored relationship. A first-place trophy is on display in our home to serve as a reminder of the new *us*.

The benefits of a revived relationship are not limited. My women's doubles partner, Karin, and I also finished the season capturing a first place trophy.

There have been more demonstrations of God's graciousness. In June our first-born, Steve, exchanged wedding vows with Sharon, a lovely, sensitive girl who shares his strong love of family and his Christian commitment. What's more, she has captivated our hearts as well, and has added a flavor of joy and creativity to our lives.

In the fall of 1979 Kim was awarded a volleyball scholarship which includes room, board, tuition, tutors and laundry service at Northwestern University. Kim is one of the first females in the university's history to be awarded a full four-year athletic scholarship for volleyball. She completed her first season as one of the starting six players on the volleyball team which went on to win the Illinois state tournament the following season, thus qualifying them to compete in the Nationals in Santa Barbara, California. Kim's number one fans, her family, also made the trip west, where Scott occupied his customary seat on the bench with the team.

In the fall of 1979, Candy shot an 83 for a first-place tie in the state single sectional golf tournament, thus qualifying for the Illinois state tournament her third consecutive year. To her father's delight, her picture appeared in the sports section of the *Chicago Tribune*. In October 1981 Candy was awarded a $750 grant by the Illinois Womens Golf Association, given to one promising golfer attending a state school in Illinois. She also received a partial golf scholarship from her school for four years. A three-sport standout in high school, Candy received varsity letters in golf, softball, and two in basketball, and was named Woman Athlete of the Year at graduation. As a freshman at Northern Illinois University, Candy was recently presented with the Most Valuable Player trophy on the women's golf team.

Thirteen year-old Scott loves learning, tennis, and working at the farm with his dad, and brother. Our combination student/farmer awakens each morning with a smile—anxious for his day to begin. Last year his family watched him win the first-place trophy in the Club's annual Junior Tennis Tournament for thirteen-year-olds and under. His pleasant personality, bright sense of humor, and keen desire for academic achievement combine to make Scott an engaging young man. In a recent letter to his Grandfather Woll, Scott wrote: "I got my report card back this week—five A's and two B's. In our school that is high honor roll. If I really had the motivation I know I could get all A's. My goal is to be Student of the Year. Please be thinking of me during these next nine weeks."

On August 3, 1980, 38 of us traveled to Lucea, Jamaica, where we conducted a Bible school for 500 Jamaicans and held 16 services in the hill country. Our only means of transportation for ten days was the back of an open sugarcane truck. Lee and I had 72 twelve-year-olds in our Bible school class who became both dear and difficult. On Friday, our final day, with the children seated in a large circle, Lee and I went slowly around the room and spoke a message of love to each child, one by one. As we looked into their eyes and held their hands in ours, soft expressions and tear-filled eyes gazed shyly back at us. At each service our singing group presented a concert of lively songs accompanied by trumpet, guitar and drums, after which Lee shared a message of God's love. Lee and I were locked in closeness as we ministered together to crowded churches. These responsive Jamaicans represented Pentecostal, Methodist, United, Catholic, Anglican, and Salvation Army denominations.

It was particularly meaningful when Lee and I knelt side by side with a row of Jamaicans in the front of the Anglican church and received communion. It was here that God changed Lee's life six years earlier and it was here that our marriage's radical recovery began. Afterwards, with tears streaking his face, Lee told the congregation of his about-face as a husband and as a total person that had begun with them.

A long-time dream has become a reality. That fall Lee and I began a book discussion group on *The Edge of Adventure* by Bruce Larson and Keith Miller. Five couples from a variety of church backgrounds endeavored to share our struggles and joys in an effort to learn more of God's purpose for our lives. At this writing we have experienced the celebration of two members making an earnest commitment to Christ as their Lord.

That June each of these couples along with their children spent a weekend camping at our farm. This occasion provided a unique opportunity for us to become better acquainted in a spectacular natural setting. We fished, canoed, hiked, swam and, by the glow of a campfire, each shared with the rest of us the year's most meaningful memory. Another highlight was a worship service held in a wooded area overlooking the river. Each family shared a specific need and then another family member prayed aloud for God to meet that need. We have decided to make it an annual tradition to invite a cluster of families to our farm to build a storehouse of lasting memories.

Our children have noticed a difference in the emotional climate of our home. To illustrate, an exerpt from a recent note from Kim: "It's good to see things are back to normal. I like seeing kissy poos when Dad comes in from work. Wow!"

And from a letter shortly after her return to campus: "I miss home very much. It was good to be able to share with you. You made the home a warm and toasty place for me to rehabilitate in after finals. I am so grateful to have such a great home to come back to. I love you guys.—Kimmy."

Today Lee and I try
—not to let disappointments determine the course of our marriage
—to take a constructive approach, concentrating on the plus features of our marriage in order to build a growing relationship based on each other's assets
—to discover common interests
—to allow each other to develop separate interests
—to stay willing to compromise
—to accept each other's need for doing his or her own thing and arrange ways for this to happen
—to permit a free flow of affection
—to limit our criticisms
—to maintain optimism and good humor
—to lower our expectations of one another
—to spend one night a week alone together—usually away from home, phone, and family interruptions

Yesterday I kept an appointment with Dr. Baker to learn whether I had a recurrence of cancer. He reaffirmed what a recent checkup with Dr. Allen had concluded:

"You are free of cancer, Janie! It has now been five glorious years and with each passing year the odds are in your favor that it will not reappear."

Date Due

2/17/85			
	PRINTED	IN U. S. A.	